5:2

VEGETARIAN

OVER 100 EASY
FASTING DIET RECIPES

CELIA BROOKS
RECIPE ANALYSIS BY ANITA BEAN

D0856171

911200000...

First published in the United Kingdom in 2013 by
PAVILION BOOKS
An imprint of Anova Books Company Ltd
10 Southcombe Street, London W14 0RA

Text © Celia Brooks
Design and layout © Anova Books 2013

The moral right of the author has been asserted

All rights reserved. No part of this work may be reproduced, or utilized in any form or by any means, electronic or mechanical, including photocopying, recording, or by any information storage and retrieval system without the prior permission of the publishers.

ISBN: 978-1-90981-501-8

A CIP record for this book is available from the British Library

10 9 8 7 6 5 4 3 2 1

Reproduction by Mission Productions Limited, Hong Kong
Printed by CPI Group (UK) Ltd, Croydon, CR0 4YY

Senior commissioning editor: Emily Preece-Morrison
Art director and cover: Georgina Hewitt
Layout: Welmoet Wartena
Editor: Maggie Ramsay
Production: Laura Brodie
Cover photograph: Clare Winfield

The information contained in this book is provided for general purposes only. It is not intended as and should not be relied upon as medical advice. The publishers and authors are not responsible for any specific health or allergy needs that may require medical supervision. If you have underlying health problems, or have any doubts about the advice contained in this book, you should consult a qualified medical, dietary, or other appropriate professional.

Notes
* Every effort has been made to give an accurate time estimate for the execution of the recipes. Where preparation techniques such as chopping are included in the method rather than the ingredients
* Cooking times are guidelines only. Where a microwave oven is used, the recipes were tested with an 800-watt microwave and cooking times may vary
* up to 3 days' mean today plus 3 days from now
* Eggs used in testing were medium size
* Authentic Parmesan is made using animal rennet. It is the responsibility of the reader to check the ingredients of any pre-processed foods to ensure that they are suitable for vegetarians if that is a concern
* This book was inspired by Dr Michael Mosley's BBC Horizon documentary Eat, Fast and Live Longer which aired in 2012. See thefastdiet.co.uk

BRENT LIBRARIES

91120000168284	
Askews & Holts	20-Dec-2013
613.25	£9.99

CONTENTS

INTRODUCTION 05

CHAPTER 1:
The 5:2 lifestyle 07

CHAPTER 2:
Essential equipment 17

CHAPTER 3:
Ingredients of the 5:2 kitchen 23

CHAPTER 4:
Easy fast-day meals 41

CHAPTER 5:
Flavour bombs 113

CHAPTER 6:
Speedy breakfasts 159

CHAPTER 7:
Simple snacks 185

CHAPTER 8:
Drinks & appetite crushers 197

CHAPTER 9:
Convenience foods & packed lunches 207

INDEX 212

ACKNOWLEDGEMENTS 221

INTRODUCTION

If you are reading this, you have just taken a step towards improving your life. If you're already a 5:2 devotee, I hope you'll embrace this book for prolonged fast-day inspiration – you know how good it feels and this is yet another step forward. If you're a newbie, what are you waiting for? You'll soon be reaping the benefits of good health, and you can start tomorrow.

So here's the scoop. The 5:2 Diet, Fast Diet, or Intermittent Fasting Diet is gaining momentum worldwide as thousands of people who try it see how effective it is for weight loss and improving their general well-being. I am one of them!

This diet emerged onto the British scene in 2012 with a BBC Horizon documentary called *Eat, Fast and Live Longer*, presented by medical journalist Dr Michael Mosley. His bestselling book *The Fast Diet* explains the science behind it. I saw the documentary in September 2012 and I decided to give 5:2 a whirl, 'fasting' for 2 days a week on 500 calories a day, and eating normally for the rest of the week.

I was quite simply blown away by how manageable it was. Four months later – and 20 pounds lighter – I started a blog about it in February 2013 called *5:2 Vegetarian*. Now I've created this book to make fast days interesting, painless and fun. On fast days, when you reduce your calorie intake by 75% just twice a week, you don't want to fuss over food – you need quick, simple and satisfying meals with a low calorie count that still taste gorgeous, so you can fit fast days into your busy life. With a little know-how, inspiration and will-power, 5:2 is the easiest diet ever – and it's easy to sustain as a lifestyle.

My message is this: **you will change with 5:2**. You'll lose weight, feel great and gain confidence. You'll drink more water and eat more vegetables, which we all know are the elixirs of life. You may find that on non-fast days your appetite is decreased and you crave more healthy foods. You also might find that you relish the foods you love even more on non-fast days. It could change your attitude to food for the better – for ever.

CHAPTER 1
THE 5:2 LIFESTYLE

Many people, me included, have found 5:2 to be effective as a weight-loss diet because it fits so easily into any lifestyle.
This is what makes it sustainable in the long term, resulting in the health benefits that are not found with conventional 'yo-yo' dieting.

WHY 5:2 VEGETARIAN?

As more 5:2-themed blogs and books spring into the public domain, many of the recipes are focused on meat and fish; they neglect the most important feature of the diet: heaps of low-calorie vegetables! Here's where I, a vegetarian food writer and 5:2 follower, am applying my expertise and creativity with vegetables. Everything here is healthy and suitable for vegetarians, with many vegan-friendly and gluten-free recipes. Eggs, tofu and beans are the main protein sources, which will help you feel fuller for longer.

Of course the book can also be enjoyed by omnivores. If you ever thought of trying a 'meatless Monday' or one day a week without meat, why not try two, and, with this book, start on a path to weight loss and better health?

The last thing you want on fast days is to be chained to the kitchen, so my fast-day meal recipes are all super-quick (30 minutes or less), satisfying, and nutrient-rich, yet all are under 300 calories. Some of the flavour bombs take a little longer to prepare, but that's only down to marinating time or time in the oven. All recipes make either one or two servings: the second portion can easily be saved for the next fast day, and most are portable, for taking to work in a packed lunch (see Chapter 9).

If you're cooking for non-fasters on fast days, I've added suggestions in Chapter 4 for multiplying and bulking out the meals for family members, as the recipes are delicious enough to share and the low-calorie aspect will go unnoticed. There are also scores of additional recipes and ideas to help on fast days, with my Flavour Bombs, Speedy Breakfasts, Snacks, Drinks and Appetite Crushers, plus a section on dressing up convenience foods and some lunchbox ideas. Now there's no excuse not to fast!

THE 5:2 DIET: HOW IT WORKS

Here's all you need to know about 5:2. The 2 refers to 2 fast days when you restrict your calorie intake to 500 for women or 600 for men on each day. The 5 refers to the rest of the week, the non-fast days, the 'feed days' or 'feast days' when you can eat normally and, within reason, enjoy all the food and drink you want. It is important not to overcompensate on these days and, as often as possible, keep it healthy. If you do over-indulge once in a while, there's no need to beat yourself up. 5:2 allows you to live life to the full.

Every weight-loss diet requires some kind of restriction on what you consume. Some diets are successful but impossible to maintain, resulting in short-term weight loss that just piles back on once you resume your normal routine. Only cabbage soup or grapefruit? Only 1000 calories every day? No chocolate, no wine, no bread, no cheese? How long can that possibly last? Not only is it excruciatingly boring and repetitive, but you feel deprived, you can't enjoy social situations, and you soon lose interest. It's simply not sustainable. Life is just too short. Even if you lose weight with one of these regimes, it soon creeps back, ounce by ounce.

The genius of 5:2 is that you need to restrict yourself only 2 days a week. It doesn't matter which days – non-consecutive or back-to-back – just whenever you can fit them into your busy week. That means you can still enjoy nights out, long lunches, or indulgent weekends with friends and family, and generally eat what you fancy, almost all week long.

By restricting yourself to the 500- or 600-calorie limit 2 days a week, you will be consuming roughly the equivalent of 3500 fewer calories per week, which equals 1 pound of fat. Once you embrace 5:2, you should lose 1 pound a week, possibly more. Fasting has other health benefits too: studies have shown that it stimulates cell repair and healing, and that it lowers your risk of diseases including heart disease, diabetes and cancer.

But I'll leave that to Dr Mosley to explain. See thefastdiet.co.uk.

MY SUCCESS STORY

My passion for food and cooking is so fervent that I made it my profession over 20 years ago. I write cookbooks, develop and demonstrate recipes, and run food tours in London. Everything I do is about inspiring people to appreciate good food. If I'm not eating or cooking it, I'm thinking about it.

Getting fat is clearly an occupational hazard for someone like me. For most of my career I've kept that hazard at bay. People often ask, 'How do you do what you do and stay slim? to which I have an automatic reply: 'tons of exercise'. I stopped hearing that question about 2 years ago. A combination of life-altering factors conspired against me and BAM! I gained 20 pounds, seemingly overnight. Carrying that extra load around marred my confidence and rendered my fabulous wardrobe obsolete. I kept beating myself up for letting it happen but I just couldn't shift it, even though I was maintaining a steady exercise regime. Then, in mid-September 2012, I stumbled across Dr Michael Mosley's BBC *Horizon* documentary online and decided to give the 5:2 discipline a try. Some weeks I cheated and, as always, I enjoyed an excessive Christmas period. Within 4 months I lost 20 pounds and have now reached my ideal weight, but I'm still keeping up with 5:2. It requires patience, but by losing weight slowly, you're more likely to keep it off. Once you achieve your goal, you'll never want to turn back. I've embraced 5:2 as a way of life, maintaining both my ideal weight and my food-loving lifestyle.

MY FAST-DAY MANTRAS

- If you're finding your fast day difficult, just remember, tomorrow you can feast!

- If you're feeling hungry but have to wait for your next meal, drink water, herbal tea or any other zero-calorie drink. Keep busy and distract yourself: do 10 jumping jacks. Call your best friend. Take out the trash. Or focus on whatever project is currently pressing. Hunger will pass.

- If you cheat or miss a fast day, don't feel guilty. It won't set you back. There's always next week to make up for it.

HOW TO BUILD YOUR BUSY LIFE AROUND 5:2

Some weeks I find it's difficult to designate 2 fast days. It's best to mark my calendar ahead of time. I try to get it over with early in the working week. I generally work from home a couple of days a week, so those are the days I choose – it's pointless trying to fast if I'm running one of my food tours or have plans for eating out. I get invited to a lot of boozy, canapé-laden industry events, so I try to schedule my fast days around those or give them a miss. I never fast at weekends, so I can be footloose and fancy-free. If I've only managed one fast day during the week, or even none, I don't beat myself up. There's always next week.

If you work outside the home all week and socialize at weekends, you'll probably need to plan your meals ahead because you really have to devote yourself to fast days. If you choose to fast during the week, you can't just load up at a salad bar or skip the bread with your soup – it's impossible to calculate the calories hidden in the food we eat outside the home, unless it's packaged and labelled. If you are at the office all day, you may find it most manageable to eat a small breakfast, bring a small snack to the office to keep you away from the biscuit tin, and skip lunch altogether, then complete your calorie allowance at home at dinnertime. Alternatively, take a fast-day friendly packed lunch to work (see pages 200–211). You'll need to choose fast days when you won't be going to a leaving-do after work or dropping round at a friend's in the evening – get yourself home and fed and it's over and you can congratulate yourself on another fast day well done.

If you're a busy parent, it can be tempting when feeding the kids to gobble down a few cheeky chips – but on fast days, don't. It may help to eat a late breakfast plus a snack, or a late lunch before they get home from school so that you aren't famished while you're cooking the kids' meal. If you eat as a family, you can expand fast-day meals to feed the non-fasters, as explained in each recipe in Chapter 4.

As for exercise, it's perfectly fine to build in your fitness on fast days, but don't overdo it, and don't compensate for extra calories burned by upping your 500- or 600-calorie allowance. You may find that you will feel extra hungry after exercise, so be prepared to stave off hunger by drinking extra water or eating your calorie-counted meal after your workout.

STRUCTURING YOUR FAST DAYS

There seem to be three different approaches to the fast day; it's just a matter of finding which system works for you:

- Literally fast all day and eat one full 500-calorie (600-calorie for men) evening meal.

- Eat breakfast and an evening meal only with nothing in between.

- Spread out three meals over the day and keep each meal under 200 calories, with the occasional snack (that's what works for me).

It does make sense to give your system a break from the constant grazing that we are accustomed to in modern life, but as far as weight loss and health benefits are concerned, it doesn't matter which configuration you choose. You'll be eating a lot less overall. You will lose weight.

There is no question that you will have some frustratingly hungry moments on fast days, but they can be overcome. Hunger waxes and wanes. If you focus on your hunger, the toys come out of the pram. Just chill. Chances are you don't have to walk more than a few feet to grab something to put in your mouth. Instead, take a walk, but not to the fridge – go outside and breathe deeply. Find distractions.

ZEN AND THE ART OF CONTROLLING HUNGER

Some people find that if they give in between meals and have a snack it makes them hungrier – after all, we are addicted to food! It's a practical discipline to just keep doing things to forget you are hungry – drinking water (or something enhanced with flavour like Fridge Tea, see page 199), keeping busy, and remembering that it will soon be over because tomorrow you can eat normally. All of these simple things help. It may also help to join one of the several online forums and Facebook groups for 5:2 to share your gripes and successes and get encouragement from others.

If you have a political or meditative nature, you might like to try mentally combatting your hunger by pondering this: how ridiculous is it that we in the Western world have been conditioned to consume constantly? Food – often the unhealthy stuff that made us fat in the first place – is all around us and we think we want it…but we don't need it, not all the time. We need good food, and we are lucky enough to be able to find it and prepare it to our liking. Consume the world around you and let it stimulate your senses – but direct your senses away from your stomach. It's only a few hours! Be Zen. You might get hungry again soon. But just settle again. This mindset gets easier with time.

Hunger focuses the mind, and it's automatic to channel that focus into becoming obsessed with being hungry. (I find this every time. I hadn't recognized this feeling until I started 5:2.) Instead, flip the switch. Use this clarity elsewhere! It's possible to be super-productive on fast days. Satiety, it seems, makes us sleepwalk through life. Fasting may affect your sleep patterns. It may also teach you about yourself and how you function in a world awash with an overabundance of edible junk.

COUNTING CALORIES AND KEEPING A CALORIE DIARY

To succeed with 5:2, you really can't make ballpark estimates about what you consume on fast days. If you are cooking with fresh ingredients, you'll need to calculate every gram and spoonful of what goes into your food. (Whenever you cook the recipes in this book, that work is done for you.) Get a comprehensive calorie-counting book, or use one of the many online calorie-counting engines – they're mostly free. You can simply search 'calories soy sauce 1 tbsp', for example, to get a result. For bulkier items such as veg, it's more accurate to measure by grams rather than 'a bunch' or 'a cup'.

Here's a system I recommend. Buy yourself a nice portable notebook for your fast-day diary or log book. Start with 'Day 1' and the date. Calculate the calories of your meals and everything else you eat and drink (if not zero-calorie) and log it in a column, with a description of what you ate.

A DAY'S EXAMPLE:

Breakfast Miso Cup (page 168)	78
Spicy Egyptian Bean Soup (page 65)	127
+ 1 tbsp low-fat yogurt	27
1 rice cake, 50g cottage cheese, alfalfa sprouts	80
One-egg Omelette (page 126)	74
+ 100g steamed broccoli	34
+ Creamy Spiked Spinach (page 136)	72
Frozen Peach & Raspberry Pop (page 194)	14
TOTAL	506

The descriptions are helpful to refer to when you are planning your fast days or wondering what to eat next, and also so you don't have to re-calculate calories as for the rice cake snack, above. This all may seem painfully tedious, but it's a system that works, and it's only two days a week. Don't count calories on non-fast days – just enjoy your food. Once you become more aware of the calorific value of food, it may alter your perception of food on non-fast days and jumpstart you into automatically eating more healthily.

You should also log in your weight every 2 to 4 fast days and watch the number shrink with relish.

MONITORING YOUR BODY WEIGHT

Before you start, you should weigh yourself and decide how much weight you want to lose. Dr Mosley recommends also getting your blood pressure, cholesterol and blood glucose levels checked by your doctor, so you can monitor the additional positive effects of 5:2. Taking a waist measurement is also a good idea.

Equip yourself with a reliable set of bathroom scales, but don't weigh yourself too often. Weigh in once a week at the most, the day after your second fast. Weigh yourself first thing in the morning and without clothes. Don't be horrified if you lose one week and gain the next: 5:2 fasters typically report weight fluctuations. Water retention and the weight of the food in your system are factors. In the long, medium or even short term, the weight will fall off. You will not keep losing weight until you disappear. At some point you will reach your ideal weight, and you can maintain 5:2 (or 6:1) to keep it that way for ever. If the weight doesn't shift, then you should look at whether you are overcompensating on non-fast days by eating more than before, or whether you aren't calculating properly, by not including what you drink, for example.

The best gauge is how your clothes fit. You may soon find yourself getting reacquainted with those favourite jeans that you thought you'd never squeeze into again. I did, along with a whole wardrobe of forgotten fashion gems – it was a thrill that made me feel confident, dynamic and 10 years younger – all achieved in about 16 weeks.

Good luck and happy fasting and feasting!

CHAPTER 2
ESSENTIAL EQUIPMENT

You'll very likely have most of the equipment discussed here. These are the tools I use on a regular basis when I'm counting calories.

KITCHEN SCALES

The most reliable way to accurately calculate the calorific value of your ingredients is by weight. Accuracy is king on fast days, because you'll want to max out your full allowance, but not go over by too much and defeat the whole exercise. Normally, I rarely bother using scales unless I am baking, which also demands accuracy. For fast-day cooking, I treat every cooking and assembly operation as if I were baking a cake, measuring out every spoonful, every gram. It goes against my bish-bash-bosh instincts, but this approach, applied just 2 days a week, allows me to keep slim – worth every tedious effort.

Any kitchen scales will do, but I use digital precision scales that measure every 2g up to 5kg. I can use any container on its flat top. When weighing vegetables for a steamed mix, for example, I'll pop a plastic or stainless-steel bowl on the scales and press the 'On Zero' button, then start chucking in a chunk of courgette, a few broccoli florets, a wedge of cabbage etc., until I reach the amount I want – say 150g. I'll then wash them and prepare as needed. (I always wash veg after weighing because the washing water clinging to the veg adds weight.) Similarly, if I need 50g of yogurt, into which I'll be stirring some other ingredients, I'll place a small mixing bowl on the scales, zero it, weigh my yogurt, then zero it again to add anything else that needs weighing, then add any other ingredients and mix it all up.

Remember, if the display seems wobbly, it's time to replace the batteries.

FREEZER

A freezer is a real advantage for storing fast-day meals. Recipes in this book suitable for freezing are identified. In general, frozen food should be used within 3 months. After that it is not dangerous (as long as it has remained frozen solid), but the flavour and texture are likely to have deteriorated.

Always allow food to cool completely before freezing, and never re-freeze thawed food. It's most space-efficient to freeze food in resealable freezer-safe bags; label them before filling. For dishes such as soups and stews, open the bag, stand it in a tall bowl, fold down the top slightly and spoon in the food, compress to let as much air out as possible and seal well before freezing. Thaw in the microwave or overnight in the fridge.

As well as a stock of resealable freezer-safe bags (large and small), you will need a permanent marker for labelling.

MICROWAVE

A microwave oven works by vibrating water molecules, thus creating heat within the food that in turn cooks it. Since most vegetables have a high water content, they lend themselves very well to being cooked in a microwave, steaming in their own juice and retaining all the valuable nutrients. For more on cooking veg in a microwave, see page 27.

Obviously microwaves are also ideal for quickly reheating food, and thawing food on the defrost setting. When reheating or defrosting, stir the food about halfway through the recommended time (protect your hands when removing a container from the microwave) and leave the food to stand for a minute or two once heated. Test that the centre of the food is piping hot before eating.

You will need microwave-safe containers for cooking. Medium-sized plastic lidded containers are best for veg – plastic take-away containers can be re-used (make sure the container is labelled as microwave-safe).

Microwave cooking and heating times vary; an 800-watt microwave was used for testing the recipes in this book.

NON-STICK FRYING PAN

This is an absolute must when you are cooking with very little fat. A good-quality 25cm/10in frying pan is the perfect size for cooking for 1 or 2. Ideally, it should also have a lid and a heatproof handle so it can be shoved under the grill (for example, for making frittatas, page 178). Choose one with a heavy bottom. When storing, do not nest pans inside it, to prevent the coating from getting scuffed. Use only wooden or non-metallic heat-proof utensils when cooking.

OTHER PANS

A lidded wok or large non-stick frying pan for stir-fries; small and medium lidded saucepans.

CALCULATOR

Essential for accurate calorie calculating.

MEASURING SPOONS AND CUPS

A good set of accurate measuring spoons is crucial: many recipes use teaspoon and tablespoon measurements, and the calories are counted for level spoonfuls.

Larger amounts are measured in jugs or cup measurements: look for a measuring jug marked in litres, fluid ounces and cups.

LEMON SQUEEZER

Fresh lemon and lime juice are essential on fast days, so how do you get the most juice out of your citrus? I can't live without a Mexican hinged 'elbow' squeezer, which extracts maximum juice in a flash and holds back seeds.

FOOD PROCESSOR AND BLENDER

Both are used occasionally in the recipes in this book. A hand-held stick blender is also useful.

MORTAR AND PESTLE

A heavy stone or rough ceramic mortar and pestle are very useful, though not essential.

FRIDGE JUG

Ideally plastic and 2-litre/3½-pint capacity with a tight-fitting lid, for water or flavoured water (see page 199).

OTHER EQUIPMENT

Tongs, scissors, garlic press, non-stick baking parchment, paper towels, and a flexible rubber spatula (for scraping out every last bit of food from your pan or food processor).

CHAPTER 3
INGREDIENTS OF
THE 5:2 KITCHEN

KNOW YOUR VEG

'Eat food. Not too much. Mostly plants.'
Michael Pollan, *In Defense of Food*

VEG: YOUR BEST FRIENDS ON FAST DAYS

After years of researching the loaded question 'What should humans eat?', author, journalist and food guru Michael Pollan boiled it down to the seven words opposite. This mantra should apply to everyday eating, and is particularly applicable on fast days. I've said it before and I'll say it again – veg are the elixir of life.

The vegetables permitted in virtually unlimited quantity on fast days are for the most part the real superheroes of the edible plant kingdom in terms of nutrition – in particular all leafy greens and brassicas (vegetables such as broccoli and cauliflower). Every vegetable has something to contribute to your health and most are low in calories but high in bulk, making them ideal fast-day fillers.

If you are not used to consuming heaps of veg on a regular basis, now is a great time to start – 2 days a week. This book is designed to help you get the best out of your veg – maximum flavour, texture and nutrition – without slaving for hours in the kitchen.

THE DEFINITIVE FAST-DAY FRESH VEG LIST

This list consists of common edible plants that can be consumed in large quantities for small calorie counts, whether eaten raw (where applicable) or steamed. The vegetables excluded from this list – potatoes, sweet potatoes, butternut squash and pumpkin, carrots, sweetcorn, peas and beans – are permitted in moderation.

alfalfa sprouts
asparagus
aubergines (eggplants)
bean sprouts
broccoli
Brussels sprouts
cabbage – all types, including kale
cauliflower
celeriac
celery
chard
chicory – all types, including Belgian
  endive, frisée, radicchio
chillies
courgettes (zucchini)
cucumbers
fennel
garlic
green beans in the pod – all types, such
  as runner (string) beans

herbs
kohlrabi
leeks
mangetout (snow peas)
mushrooms – all types, cultivated
  and wild
onions – all types
pak choi (bok choy)
peppers
radishes
salad leaves – all types
seed sprouts – all types, such as
  alfalfa, cress
spinach
sugar-snap peas
swede (rutabaga)
tomatoes
turnips

SELECTING VEG

Of course fresh is always best, and if you are keeping recipe portions for up to 3 days, it is vital that you start with the freshest ingredients possible. But just how fresh are the veg you buy in a supermarket? As soon as a vegetable stops growing, it starts losing flavour and nutrient value, so if you can get your veg from a farmer's market or organic box scheme, you will be cutting out middle men and thus time for it to start dying. Better still, if you are lucky enough to have a garden or allotment, grow your own.

PREPARING VEG

As a general rule, it's best to prepare veg when you need them rather than buying ready-prepared, for the best flavour and freshness. I cheat on this rule with spinach – I buy bags of ready-washed baby spinach so that I can easily grab a large handful to stir into soups and stews just before serving. Weigh your veg before washing and preparing, as washing water will register on the scales.

STORING VEG

Almost all veg are best stored in the fridge in sealed plastic bags (though mushrooms keep better in paper bags) in the designated drawers, which maintain moisture and prevent damage from contact with the fridge walls. Garlic, ginger and regular onions should be kept in a cool dry place. Even potatoes, I find, keep longer in the fridge, though some swear by storing them like onions. Keep cut veg (for example, half a pepper or courgette) in a resealable bag or airtight container in the fridge and use within 3 days. Your nose will be the best judge as to whether your stored veg is still OK to use, but chuck any that show signs of over-softness or sliminess.

COOKING VEG

On fast days, veg from the list opposite should be steamed to maintain nutrients, and that is most easily and quickly done in the microwave (see page 19). Place your prepared veg in a microwave-safe container, add a sprinkle of water (1–2 tsp) and a pinch of salt if desired, then cover. Microwaves vary, but a rough guide is to cook on high power for 1 minute per 50g, then stand for about 30 seconds. Protect your hands when taking the container from the microwave, and be careful when removing the lid, as the steam is scorchingly hot. Save any cooking juices in the container and add to your food, or cool slightly and gulp them down as a hot health tonic with no calories.

PULSES AND OTHER VEG

- **Beans:** Along with tofu (see page 31) and eggs, beans are the vegetarian's go-to low-fat protein source. Canned beans of all types (without added sauce) are acceptable, as are cooked beans in cartons. Always drain and rinse the beans first, then weigh for the recipe. Unused beans can be stored in the fridge in an airtight container (not in the can) for up to 3 days and can also be frozen.

- **Refried beans:** These are not actually fried at all, but are mashed pinto beans with spices, perfect for Mexican-style meals such as Breakfast Burrito (page 182) and low in calories as long as they are fat-free. Seek out half-size cans and store unused portions as for beans, above.

- **Lentils:** Lentils of all sorts are good for fast days. Puy lentils, black and brown lentils are hugely flavourful and can be found ready-cooked in cans, pouches or cartons. From dried, red lentils cook the fastest, in 15–20 minutes.

- **Artichoke hearts:** A fast-day favourite at just 30 cals per 100g. Choose hearts in brine rather than oil. Frozen hearts and artichoke bottoms are also available. Store unused portions as for beans, above.

- **Palm hearts:** Also labelled as hearts of palm, these are a fabulous raw or cooked ingredient with a wonderful flavour and a creamy texture, and just 31 cals per 100g. I often munch them straight out of the can. Store unused portions as for beans, above.

- **Tomatoes:** Canned Italian chopped or whole peeled tomatoes in juice and cherry tomatoes in juice are an ideal convenience food for fast-day recipes. Passata (strained tomatoes), usually sold in a jar or carton, is also a staple – check the label to make sure no oil or sugar has been added.

- **Pickled veg:** All pickles are brilliant for fast days, as they have very few calories and bags of taste and texture: use them in salads, for general plate-expanding, and snacking. Choose pickles without any added sugar or oil and stock up on cucumbers/gherkins, beetroot, jalapeño peppers, onions, garlic, cabbage, or any others you fancy.

- **Sauerkraut:** A satisfying, virtually calorie-free snack and a useful ingredient too, it's also packed with beneficial bacteria from the lactic fermentation for an added health boost.

- **Frozen veg:** Peas, sweetcorn, and broad beans all feature in this book. Frozen broccoli is good to have on hand for emergencies in case you suddenly find your fresh veg drawer is empty on a fast day.

FRUIT

Fresh fruit contains fructose, a sugar, which has an impact on insulin, the hormone produced by the body to regulate blood sugar levels. The higher your blood sugar, the more insulin is produced; an hour or so later, the insulin and blood sugar levels drop rapidly, making you feel even more hungry. Berries, stone fruits (cherries, plums, peaches, etc.), grapes, apples, pears and figs are the best choices, but gram for gram are considerably higher in calories than most veg. However, all fruits contain beneficial nutrients and, naturally, they're delicious – I have used mango and pineapple in some savoury recipes. Frozen grapes on a stick are a good fast-day snack.

OTHER STAPLE INGREDIENTS

The huge array of fresh, canned and
frozen vegetables discussed in the
preceeding pages will be your fast-day
heroes. But to conjure up truly exciting
low-cal meals in double-quick time, you'll
need to stock up on a variety of protein
sources and ingredients for creating high-
impact flavour, both fresh and long-life.

FRESH STAPLES

TOFU

The high protein and low fat content of tofu make it ideal for filling you up and keeping you full on fast days. It's a brilliant receptor of flavour, welcoming high-impact sauces and marinades.

Seasoned vegetarians will be familiar with this essential protein source, but some don't really enjoy eating tofu, because in its natural, naked state, it's undeniably bland. The fact is, it needs a boost to make it truly tasty, such as immersion in a flavourful marinade and/or frying, grilling or baking to provide texture. Frying tofu gives it a delicious crisp skin, but adds a lot of high-calorie oil, so this cooking method is largely ignored in this book. However, tofu can be roasted or lightly fried in minimal oil to great effect, as in Teriyaki Tofu & Roasted Broccoli (page 99) or Classic Stir-Fry with Tofu (page 71).

Buying tofu:
- Buy fresh tofu labelled as 'firm'. Long-life tofu, even if labelled 'firm', has a custardy texture, which is difficult to work with and falls apart easily.

- The calorie content of tofu varies quite a lot, so try to find one that clocks in around 76 cals per 100g.

- Smoked tofu has a higher calorie content per 100g than fresh because it has lost water weight in the smoking process and is more dense. It has a great flavour, but you will have to reduce the quantity in the recipes to meet the correct calorie count.

- Ready-marinated tofu will usually be too calorific for fast days, so save it for other days.

Using and storing tofu:
- Use scissors to release the tofu from its watery packaging, holding it over the sink. Drain well and wrap in paper towels, pressing gently to absorb

as much excess liquid as possible. Next, weigh out the required amount for the recipe.

- The remainder can be stored in the fridge for up to 3 days – place in an airtight container or resealable bag and add a little fresh water. If possible, change the water daily.

- Tofu can also be frozen. Label a resealable freezer bag, writing the date and weight of the tofu. Cut the patted-dry tofu into cubes, place in the bag, seal well, expelling as much air as possible, and freeze for up to 3 months. Because of the high water content, ice crystals will form during freezing, which alters the texture of the tofu, making it slightly chewy and fibrous – dare I say, a little like chicken! Some people prefer it this way to the fresh, creamy curds. To use from frozen, simply weigh out what you need from the freezer, place it in a small bowl or cup and pour boiling water over it. Stand for 5 minutes, then drain, pat dry and use as fresh in the recipe.

MISO

This delicious savoury paste is most familiar when diluted as a soup, but it can also be used as an ingredient, imparting a salty umami flavour and boosting protein intake. There are many different types, ranging from very pale 'white miso' to almost black – the darker the colour, the stronger and saltier the taste. It is usually found in the chiller section in Asian markets and health food shops, though long-life versions are available from supermarkets; these should be refrigerated after opening and used within about 4–6 weeks – check the label.

One tbsp of miso paste has roughly 30 cals. Some miso is made using wheat or barley in the fermentation process, so check the label if you need it to be gluten-free.

Sachets of powdered miso soup are also a great fast-day standby and can be enjoyed plain or as a soup stock.

EGGS

Nature's perfect protein, at about 74 cals per egg, the egg is a superhero for fast-day satiety. Buy organic if possible and free-range unquestionably. Store in the fridge.

Hard-boiled eggs are very handy for fast-day salads and recipes so it's good to boil 2 or 3 at a time and keep them refrigerated, in the shell, for up to a week. I prefer mine 'butter-yolked' rather than rock-hard and powdery – that is, the yolk is set throughout but the very centre has a creamy consistency. To achieve this, I use the following method: cover eggs in cold water, bring to the boil, simmer for 7 minutes, drain and rinse until cold. This timing works for medium eggs, which were used for testing the recipes.

CHEESE

Real, freshly grated Parmesan (Parmigiano Reggiano) contributes a lot of flavour for its mere 22 cals per tbsp. However, genuine Parmesan is always made using animal rennet, so if you are a strict vegetarian, you may choose to substitute or leave it out. There are some very respectable Parmesan-style cheeses that use vegetarian rennet, so seek them out. Finely grate your own for the best flavour, though fresh ready-grated Parmesan is a good stand-by if you're in a hurry. Dried (not fresh) Italian Parmesan-style powdered cheese is best avoided, though it may have a certain nostalgic appeal to some. Other cheeses that are useful for fast days include cottage cheese, light cream cheese, reduced-fat feta and low-fat cheese spread (in tubs or 15g triangles) – check the label to ensure they are suitable for vegetarians.

LEMONS AND LIMES

You'll be getting through a lot of these! They'll keep the longest if stored in a sealed bag in the fridge. You'll get roughly 2 tbsp of juice from 1 lemon, possibly less from a lime – limes are sometimes tough to squeeze, so buy extra. I have specified either lemon or lime juice in the recipes and sometimes both; the two juices are interchangeable.

CUPBOARD STAPLES

- **Shirataki noodles**: Also referred to as 'zero noodles' or 'miracle noodles', these are a godsend on fast days and provide the perfect base for many recipes in this book in lieu of pasta or grains. What's so great about them? They contain virtually no calories or carbs in a substantial serving. They are a natural product derived from a root called konjac and have been used in Asia for years. They come in long-life packets (from health food shops and online) and appear ready-to-eat, but they definitely need a bit of attention before you consume them. It is very important to follow the cooking instructions on page 116 to make them palatable. They come in classic 'ramen noodle' form and also in 'rice' form (which is just the noodles snipped into tiny pieces) and other 'pasta' shapes. All are flavourless in themselves, but absorb flavours well and are a good source of dietary fibre and a brilliant stomach-filler.

- **Oils**: A spray oil or cooking spray is indispensable for fast days, delivering just the minimum of lubrication for cooking quickly and effectively. Sunflower oil is good for high-temperature cooking (such as stir-fries); extra-virgin olive oil is good for salads and gentle cooking. My first choice of oil for all cooking and salads is extra-virgin or cold-pressed rapeseed oil – it tastes nutty, can be used at all temperatures and is a good source of omega 3s. All oils have about 40 cals per tsp, so are used very sparingly on fast days. A small amount of butter or margarine is also used for cooking eggs and occasionally smearing on toast.

- **Salt**: I use sea salt flakes mostly for seasoning, using fingertips to crush it pinch by pinch into food. Table salt is used in larger quantities to season water for boiling noodles, potatoes, etc.

- **Vegetable stock**: Soups feature prominently in this book, so good stock is a necessity, but I'm not one to insist on always making fresh stock. Vegetable stock powder or cubes are perfectly acceptable. If you can, save the water used for steaming, boiling or microwaving veg and either add to food, drink it as a hot tonic, or cool, bag and freeze it for stock.

- **Soy sauce**: Both light and dark soy sauce are essential in the 5:2 kitchen. Teriyaki sauce is another tasty condiment for flavouring steamed veg, noodles, tofu and soups, but check the label for calories as some contain rather a lot of sugar. If you need to eat gluten-free, check that the soy sauce is suitable, as some contain wheat.

- **Vinegars**: Splash out on the finest vinegars you can afford: balsamic, red wine, white wine and cider vinegar – good-quality vinegar delivers way more flavour than acidity alone, for next to zero calories. Sushi vinegar or seasoned rice vinegar has a little sugar and salt added (about 7 cals per tsp), but is a wonderful flavour booster for many recipes or simply used on its own as a salad dressing.

- **Chilli**: You may notice from my recipes that I love spicy food! Chilli not only starts a party in your mouth but it speeds up your metabolism, so it's a fast-day superstar. Leave it out if you're not a fan; otherwise, stock up on dried chilli flakes, cayenne pepper, hot chilli sauces such as Tabasco (a little goes a long way for 0 cals) and a garlicky Thai sauce such as Sriracha (6 cals per tsp), pickled jalapeños, and of course fresh chillies – small ones pack a punch and can be stored in the freezer. Thaw frozen chillies under warm water for a few seconds to soften, then snip with scissors directly into the food, rather than risking getting the stinging juice on your hands by chopping on a board.

- **Spices**: My fast-day heroes are: freshly ground black pepper, cumin (seeds and ground), cinnamon, nutmeg (store whole and grate when needed), Hungarian paprika, Spanish smoked paprika (pimentón), saffron strands, turmeric, fennel seeds and coriander seeds. I also use spice mixes such as curry powder or garam masala, chat masala for sprinkling on cucumbers and fruit, ras-el-hanout (a Moroccan spice mix) and taco seasoning or a Mexican-style chilli powder mix. Store spices in tightly closed jars or tins out of the light – I store mine in a deep kitchen drawer – spice racks are certain death for spices. Don't use ground spices if they don't smell pungent – using anything over about 2 years old will be the equivalent of adding dust to your food.

- **Herbs**: I use a lot of dried dill – I'm a big dill fan but don't always have it fresh to hand – it's brilliant with eggs and lots more besides. Dried thyme, oregano and dried mixed Italian-style herbs are always useful. Buy fresh herbs as you need them and store in sealed bags in the fridge. Keep a basil plant year-round in the kitchen – pinch off the tips as needed to keep the plant flourishing.

- **Garlic and garlic powder**: Fresh garlic is usually crushed before use in recipes, but first, I always inspect each clove for a sprout and remove it, especially if I'm using it raw, as it can have an unpleasant flavour. I've recently embraced garlic powder or granules – this is extremely useful to grab off the shelf to add garlic flavour in a hurry. I used to turn my nose up at this stuff, but it's a godsend on fast days.

- **Ginger**: I always use fresh ginger in recipes and also infused in boiling water for tea as a digestive tonic. Use the tip of a teaspoon to peel it easily, or if the recipe calls for a specific amount, such as 'a 1cm piece', cut the required amount, then lay it cut-side down and slice downward, close to the edge, to cut off the skin, then chop or grate as required.

- **Sweeteners**: As a healthier alternative to refined white sugar, I use small amounts of agave nectar or honey to perk up savoury dishes. Since such a small amount is used, not too many calories are gained at 20 cals per tsp. When a stronger sweetness is needed, for example for sweetening drinks or porridge, I resort to ultra-low-cal sugar substitutes with close to zero calories: Truvia®, made from the stevia plant, is my usual choice. Canderel Green® or Splenda® are other options.

- **Sweet cooking wines**: These include Madeira, Marsala, sherry and vin santo; for the purposes of this book, they are interchangeable as very little is needed for flavouring. Mirin (Japanese sweet rice wine) and Shaoxing or Shaoshing (the Chinese equivalent) are the best choices for Asian-style dishes, but sherry or others can be substituted.

- **Dried mushrooms**: Shiitake and porcini are my flavouring favourites. When soaked in hot water or boiled, they impart a rich flavour to the liquid. The mushrooms themselves are restored to a toothsome version of their original fresh selves – perfect for adding depth and texture to soups and stews.

- **Sesame seeds**: Toasting sesame seeds really brings out their nutty flavour – sprinkle on salads, veg and noodle dishes. To toast them, heat a small frying pan over a medium–high heat (no oil), add the raw sesame seeds and stir attentively until golden and popping. Remove from the pan and tip onto a plate to cool, then use or store. Though freshly toasted sesame seeds are best, I've taken to toasting a small (about 50g) batch and storing them in an airtight container; they keep for about 2 weeks. They are high-calorie but nutritious, and contribute way more flavour than their tiny size suggests. Calculate 17 cals per tsp or 52 cals per tbsp.

- **Nuts**: Walnut pieces and flaked almonds are used in moderation, for protein, flavour and crunch. All nuts can be stored in the freezer for optimum freshness.

- **Mustard**: Hot English and Dijon mustard provide a big hit of flavour for very few calories.

- **Capers and olives**: Buy them in brine and store in the fridge once open.

- **Salsa**: Mexican-style salsa is usually fat-free and around 27 cals per 100g, so it can be used freely as a punchy flavour boost, or as a snack with celery sticks.

- **Protein powder**: Adding protein is a good thing on fast days, as it increases your feeling of fullness. Protein powder (available from health food shops) can be added to smoothies or sprinkled over yogurt or porridge, but do take the calories into account – check the label.

- **Xanthan gum**: Use just a tiny amount to thicken smoothies – for more info see page 164.

SOME HEALTHY FOODS YOU WON'T FIND IN THIS BOOK…

- **Avocado**: One delicious, nutritious avocado will set you back nearly 300 calories: 284 cals for 1 medium avocado.

- **Hummus**: Standard hummus is loaded with olive oil and tahini (sesame seed paste, which is also high in oil) and is best saved for feast days. Seek out low-calorie versions if you like, but they're still quite high in calories and far inferior to the rich and yummy original.

- **Nuts**: Not the wisest choice for a low-cal snack, though I use nuts in some recipes.

- **Peanut butter**: 1 tbsp will cost you about 95 cals – almost 20% of your fast-day allowance.

- **Wholegrains**: While I do recommend and use some wholegrains, there are lower-calorie options, such as Cauliflower Couscous (page 118).

CHAPTER 4
EASY FAST-DAY MEALS

ON FAST DAYS, you probably don't want to prepare labour-intensive food, but you still want to enjoy it, which is why I've created these easy, quick, low-cal recipes. All can be made in 30 minutes or less, and all have fewer than 300 calories per serving. Chances are that you are the only one in your household on a fast day – or perhaps you're sharing with one other person. So here's my design for this chapter:

- All recipes make 1 or 2 servings.

- All recipes for 2 servings are designed so that the second serving can be kept until the next fast day, or frozen – full storage info is given.

- All recipes can be easily and reliably multiplied to feed a family – suggestions for family meal accompaniments (for those not fasting) are made at the bottom of the recipe ('Feed the non-fasters'), so you don't have to cook separately for yourself every time.

- All recipes have calorie counts under 300 cals per serving (most are well under).

- Fast-friendly additions with calorie counts are included.

BROAD BEAN & BASIL PURÉE PLATTER

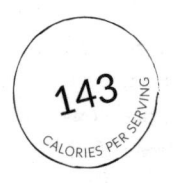

143 CALORIES PER SERVING

Gluten-free

NUTRITIONAL INFO PER SERVING: 1g fat, of which 0.4g saturates

19g carbohydrate, of which 5g sugars \\ 14g protein \\ 0.1g salt \\ 13g fibre

---

This fresh, bright-green cousin of hummus just cries out to be dipped into. Assemble your platter with a selection of crunchy crudités and other tasty morsels from the list below, according to your calorie allowance. Even if you are a stickler for peeling broad beans, rest assured this is completely unnecessary here – the bean skins contribute a lovely chewy texture plus extra nutritional value and fibre.

PREP & COOK TIME: **15 MINUTES**

SERVINGS: **2 LARGE**

300g/10½oz/2 cups frozen broad (fava) beans

1 garlic clove

2 tbsp fresh lemon juice

large handful (about 10g/¼oz) of fresh basil, or 12 large tips

2 tbsp low-fat yogurt

sea salt and freshly ground black pepper

Accompaniments

raw vegetables cut into dippable pieces: cucumber, celery, carrots, fennel, broccoli, cauliflower, red or green peppers, Little Gem lettuce leaves (20–40 cals per 100g)

rye or melba toast crackers (check the label for calories)

1 hard-boiled egg (72 cals)

pickled onions and gherkins (23 cals per 100g)

1 Bring a small saucepan of water to the boil and add the broad beans and the garlic. Bring to the boil and then reduce the heat and simmer until the beans are tender, about 3–4 minutes.

2 | Grab a container to collect the cooking liquid and drain the beans over it, reserving the garlic with the beans. Leave to cool for a couple of minutes.

3 | Put the beans and garlic in a food processor with the lemon juice, basil, yogurt, salt and pepper, plus 8 tbsp of the cooking liquid (the rest can be saved for soup stock). Process at high speed, scraping down the sides now and then, until as smooth as possible. Taste for seasoning and whizz in more salt or lemon juice if necessary.

4 | Serve while warm, or serve chilled.

\\ Keep in an airtight container in the fridge for up to 3 days. Can also be frozen; thaw completely and stir thoroughly before serving.

RAW CAULIFLOWER & FETA TABBOULEH

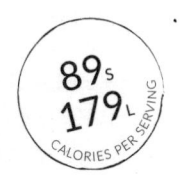

89s
179L
CALORIES PER SERVING

Gluten-free \\ Dairy-free \\ Vegan (if the feta is replaced with walnuts)
NUTRITIONAL INFO PER SERVING: (1 large serving) 9g fat, of which 3g saturates
11g carbohydrate, of which 10g sugars \\ 14g protein \\ 0.8g salt \\ 7g fibre

Inspired by my discovery of Cauliflower Couscous (page 118) – which, as a base for hot dishes, is best served lightly steamed in place of a grain – I decided to try it raw, in place of bulgur wheat for tabbouleh, and here is the extremely pleasing result. I've included reduced-fat feta cheese for protein; add 37 cals if using regular feta. Chopped walnuts could be substituted for the feta.

PREP TIME: **15 MINUTES**
SERVINGS: **2 SMALL OR 1 LARGE**

150g/5½oz cauliflower florets
1 unwaxed lemon
1 tsp extra-virgin rapeseed oil or
  olive oil
sea salt and freshly ground
  black pepper

25g/1oz cucumber
6 cherry tomatoes
2 spring onions (scallions)
large handful of fresh parsley
large handful of fresh mint
25g/1oz reduced-fat feta cheese

1 Put the cauliflower in the food processor and whizz at high speed until reduced to tiny granules, then scrape into a bowl.

2 Wash the lemon well and finely grate the zest over the bowl of cauliflower – the outer layer only, no pith. Squeeze the juice and add 1 tbsp to the bowl, then add the oil. Season generously with salt and pepper, stir well and set aside.

3 Roughly chop the cucumber, slice or quarter the tomatoes and slice the spring onions. Strip the parsley and mint from the stems and chop finely (if saving the second portion for another day, keep the mint separate and chop or tear into the mixture just before serving). Mix the veg and herbs through the cauliflower.

4 Crumble the feta into the mixture and stir well, then serve.

\\ If desired, serve on a bed of young salad leaves or in Little Gem lettuce cups.

\\ Keep in an airtight container in the fridge for up to 3 days; keep the mint separate and add it fresh just before serving so it doesn't discolour. Not suitable for freezing.

\\ Feed the non-fasters: multiply ingredients as necessary and serve with bread and hummus.

CREAMY POTATO & EGG SALAD

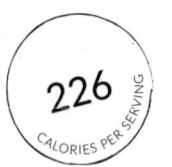

226 CALORIES PER SERVING

Gluten-free

NUTRITIONAL INFO PER SERVING: 8g fat, of which 3g saturates
23g carbohydrate, of which 9g sugars \\ 15g protein \\ 1.2g salt \\ 2g fibre

---

Here's one seriously substantial salad. The dressing alone (69 cals) is suitable for all manner of fresh salad items, though it particularly loves the company of potatoes, eggs and leaves. Consider adding pickled or fresh boiled or grated raw beetroot, or grated carrots or celeriac.

PREP & COOK TIME: **20 MINUTES**
SERVINGS: **1 LARGE**

100g/3½oz new or salad potatoes
sea salt and freshly ground
    black pepper
1 egg
mixed salad leaves such as rocket
    (arugula), watercress, romaine hearts,
    baby spinach

Dressing
1 medium pickled cucumber
1 spring onion (scallion)
handful of fresh herbs, such as dill,
    mint, parsley, chives
100g/3½oz/scant ½ cup low-fat yogurt
1 tsp Dijon mustard
1–2 tsp wine vinegar or vinegar from
    the pickle jar

1   Cut the potatoes into bite-sized pieces. Place in a small pan, cover with cold water and add salt. Place the egg in another small pan and cover with cold water. Place both pans over a high heat and bring to the boil. Once boiling, reduce the heat to a simmer. Set the timer for 7 minutes.

2   For the dressing, chop the pickle, onion and herbs. Stir into the yogurt and add the mustard, vinegar, salt and pepper. Stir and taste for seasoning.

3 Arrange the salad leaves on a plate.

4 When the timer dings, take the egg off the heat and rinse under cold water until cool. Check the potatoes for tenderness; drain well once cooked through.

5 Peel the egg and cut into quarters. Arrange on the salad leaves. Add the potato and smother with the creamy dressing.

\\ Keep the cooked, cooled potatoes, boiled egg (in shell) and dressing in separate airtight containers in the fridge for up to 3 days. Not suitable for freezing.

SPICY PALM HEART & EGG SALAD

129 CALORIES PER SERVING

Gluten-free \\ Dairy-free
NUTRITIONAL INFO PER SERVING: 7g fat, of which 2g saturates
7g carbohydrate, of which 3g sugars \\ 9g protein \\ 0.2g salt \\ 3g fibre

Palm hearts and eggs are the best of friends (see also Palm Heart Scramble, page 177), and here they pair up in a filling summery salad with a cumin- and chilli-laced dressing. Make sure you use very fresh cumin for this, not a spoonful of dust from the back of the cupboard. For best results, use about ¾ tsp cumin seeds and crush them to a rough powder in a mortar or spice grinder, then the flavour will sing! I've made suggestions for the green salad base here, but use what you have available within 5:2 parameters (page 26).

PREP & COOK TIME: **20 MINUTES**

SERVINGS: **2 LARGE**

2 eggs
200g/7oz canned palm hearts
   (approx. 1 can, drained)
2 tbsp fresh lime juice
½ tsp ground cumin
¼ tsp cayenne pepper
½ tsp agave nectar or honey
1 tsp olive oil
sea salt and freshly ground
   black pepper

Salad greens

100g/3½oz baby salad leaves
50g/1¾oz cucumber, sliced
1 spring onion (scallion) or a few chives,
   sliced or snipped
handful of alfalfa or radish sprouts
a few fresh mint and/or parsley leaves

1. Place the eggs in a pan and cover with cold water. Bring to the boil, reduce the heat and simmer for 7 minutes. Drain and refresh under cold water, then peel and cut into quarters. (If saving the second portion, keep the second egg in the shell and refrigerate.)

2. Meanwhile, slice the palm hearts quite thickly.

3. Whisk together the lime juice, cumin, cayenne, agave or honey, olive oil, salt and pepper. Taste and adjust the seasoning.

4. Arrange your salad greens on a plate and top with palm hearts and egg quarters. Spoon over the dressing and serve. (If saving the second portion, use half the dressing and refrigerate the rest.)

\\ Add a little extra flavour and nutrition by sprinkling with toasted sesame seeds (52 cals per tbsp).

\\ Keep the boiled egg (in shell), sliced palm hearts and dressing in separate airtight containers in the fridge for up to 3 days. Not suitable for freezing.

THAI SALAD WRAPS WITH CHARGRILLED TOFU

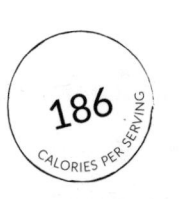

186 CALORIES PER SERVING

Gluten-free (if gluten-free soy sauce is used) \\ Dairy-free \\ Vegan

NUTRITIONAL INFO PER SERVING: 8g fat, of which 1g saturates

16g carbohydrate, of which 15g sugars \\ 12g protein \\ 4.1g salt \\ 5g fibre

Turnips, swede and kohlrabi are all members of the cabbage family and are rich in cancer-fighting phytonutrients as well as being super-low in calories, but these veg are often overlooked. When grated raw into salads, they absorb flavours beautifully and deliver a light and fresh flavour of their own which marries well with this sweet, sour and hot dressing. Grab whichever one you can get your hands on: turnips, though available year-round, are best in spring and summer; kohlrabi is best from July to November; and swede throughout the winter until April.

PREP & COOK TIME: **30 MINUTES**

SERVINGS: **2 LARGE**

1 tbsp sesame seeds

200g/7oz fresh firm tofu

150g/5½oz turnip, kohlrabi or swede (rutabaga)

½ red pepper

50g/1¾oz green beans

2 spring onions (scallions)

handful of fresh mint leaves

spray oil

4 round lettuce leaves

Dressing

1 garlic clove

1 or 2 small red or green chillies, to taste

3 tbsp light soy sauce

2 tbsp fresh lime juice

1 tbsp agave nectar or honey

1 | Heat a non-stick frying pan over a medium–high heat. Add the sesame seeds and cook, stirring frequently, until golden and popping. Remove the seeds to a plate to cool.

2 | Drain the tofu and wrap in paper towels. Set aside.

3 | For the dressing, peel the garlic and remove any sprout. Ideally, use a mortar and pestle: snip in the chilli, add the garlic and pound until smashed, then add the soy sauce, lime juice and agave or honey, and blend well with the pestle. Alternatively, crush the garlic and chop the chilli and combine with the remaining dressing ingredients in a bowl, mixing well.

4 | Peel and grate the turnip, kohlrabi or swede on the coarse side of a cheese grater. Slice the pepper thinly. Top the beans and slice them and the onions thinly on the diagonal. Combine the veg thoroughly in a bowl, reserving the mint leaves. Reserve 1 tbsp of the dressing, then stir the rest through the salad and set aside. (If saving the second portion, keep half the dressing separate and cook the tofu just before serving.)

5 | Heat a ridged grill pan over a high heat. Cut the tofu into 1cm/½in-thick slabs and spray each side with oil. Chargrill on each side until deep golden stripes appear – use a fork to turn the tofu.

6 | Meanwhile, assemble the salad. Lay 2 lettuce leaves on each plate and top with the salad mixture. Scatter over the mint leaves and sprinkle with toasted sesame seeds.

7 | Top each wrap with a piece of tofu, spoon the reserved dressing over the tofu, and serve.

\\ Keep the dressing, mint, lettuce and sesame seeds in separate airtight containers in the fridge for up to 3 days. Cook the tofu just before serving. Not suitable for freezing.

\\ Feed the non-fasters: Multiply ingredients as necessary. Serve with egg noodles dressed with light soy sauce, or rice cooked in half water, half coconut milk.

MANGO & BLACK BEAN SALAD

Gluten-free \\ Dairy-free \\ Vegan (if the dressing is omitted)
NUTRITIONAL INFO PER SERVING: 1g fat, of which 0.1g saturates
25g carbohydrate, of which 8g sugars \\ 9g protein \\ 0.6g salt \\ 11g fibre
WITH DRESSING: 2g fat, of which 0.5g saturates \\ 29g carbohydrate, of which 11g
sugars \\ 11g protein \\ 0.7g salt \\ 11g fibre

This South American-inspired salad combines to form a winning balance of texture, flavour, colour and healthfulness. Use ready-prepared fresh mango or peel a fresh one. There's plenty of deliciousness going on already, but if you have time to stir 4 ingredients together, the Cumin-Yogurt Dressing is a fabulous addition (this sauce is also used in Spanish Stir-fry, page 72).

PREP & COOK TIME: **15 MINUTES**
SERVINGS: **2 LARGE**

240g/8½oz/1 cup canned black beans
  (1 x 400g can, drained)
2 tbsp fresh lime juice
sea salt and freshly ground
  black pepper
2 spring onions (scallions)
1 large red chilli

50g/1¾oz frozen sweetcorn
100g/3½oz prepared fresh mango
handful of fresh mint leaves or fresh
  coriander (cilantro)

Cumin-Yogurt Dressing (optional)
100g/3½oz/scant ½ cup low-fat yogurt
½ tsp ground cumin
2 tsp fresh lime or lemon juice .
sea salt

1 Rinse the black beans thoroughly and drain them well. Place in a bowl and add the lime juice and plenty of seasoning.

2 Chop the spring onions. Deseed and chop the chilli, then stir through the beans.

3. Put the sweetcorn in a microwave-safe container and cook on high power until tender, about 1 minute. Drain and rinse under cold water until cool. Add to the beans and stir.

4. Cut the mango into small pieces and chop the mint, then stir through the beans. Serve, or add the dressing.

5. To make the dressing, simply stir everything together, season to taste, and spoon over the beans.

\\ Enjoy on its own or on a bed of salad leaves, or with a baked sweet potato.

\\ Keep in the fridge for up to 3 days, provided that the mango is not already overly ripe. Keep the mint separate and add it fresh just before serving so it doesn't discolour. Keep the Cumin-Yogurt dressing separate, if using. Not suitable for freezing.

\\ Feed the non-fasters: Multiply ingredients as necessary and drizzle with extra-virgin olive oil.

BLACK-EYED PEA & COCONUT SALAD

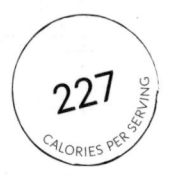

227 CALORIES PER SERVING

Gluten-free \\ Dairy-free \\ Vegan
NUTRITIONAL INFO PER SERVING: 7g fat, of which 7g saturates
25g carbohydrate, of which 3g sugars \\ 12g protein \\ 1.3g salt \\ 9g fibre

Black-eyed peas or beans have a distinctive nutty flavour. As with any bean, they are a welcome fast-day protein injection, and here they are elevated with an exotic Asian-style treatment. The coconut is a bit naughty in the calorie department, but is extremely filling and complementary to the beans.

PREP & COOK TIME: **15 MINUTES**
SERVINGS: **2 LARGE**

25g/1oz/4 tbsp unsweetened
  desiccated coconut
2 tbsp boiling water
215g/7½oz/1¼ cups canned black-
  eyed peas (1 x 400g can, drained)

100g/3½oz cucumber
2 spring onions (scallions)
2 tbsp fresh lime juice
1 tsp agave nectar or honey
½ tsp ground cumin
½ tsp salt, or to taste
small handful of fresh mint

1 Boil the kettle. Put the coconut in a small bowl and add the 2 tbsp boiling water. Leave for about 10 minutes to plump and soften.

2 Meanwhile, drain and rinse the beans. Dice the cucumber and slice the spring onions. Combine in a bowl.

3 To the bowl of coconut, add the lime juice, agave or honey, cumin and salt, and stir well. Add to the bean mixture and combine thoroughly.

4 Strip the mint leaves from their stalks and chop coarsely, then stir through the salad and serve. (Note: if saving the second portion, save half the unchopped mint to stir through just before serving.)

\\ Enjoy on its own or on a bed of mixed salad leaves.

\\ Keep in an airtight container in the fridge for up to 3 days; keep the mint separate so it doesn't discolour, and chop into the salad just before serving. Not suitable for freezing.

\\ Feed the non-fasters: Multiply ingredients as necessary and drizzle with extra-virgin olive oil. Serve with baked or buttered mashed sweet potato.

MICRO-BROCCOLI SALAD WITH SWEET SEED CLUSTERS & EGG

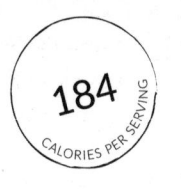
184 CALORIES PER SERVING

Gluten-free \\ Dairy-free
NUTRITIONAL INFO PER SERVING: 12g fat, of which 2g saturates
6g carbohydrate, of which 5g sugars \\ 12g protein \\ 0.2g salt \\ 3g fibre

---

This is a slightly eccentric salad, but it really is delicious. Ordinary broccoli is blitzed in the food processor to a crumb-like consistency (hence 'micro'), and is eaten raw. Combined with the protein-rich boiled egg and sunflower seeds, this makes a really filling and über-healthy superfood salad.

PREP & COOK TIME: **20 MINUTES**
SERVINGS: **2 MEDIUM**

2 eggs
2 tbsp sunflower seeds
  (about 20g/¾oz)
1 tsp agave nectar or honey

sea salt and freshly ground
  black pepper
150g/5½oz broccoli
1 tbsp fresh lemon juice
1 tsp extra-virgin rapeseed oil or
  olive oil

1 Place the eggs in a small pan and cover with cold water. Bring to the boil, reduce the heat and simmer for 7 minutes. Drain and run under cold water until cool.

2 Meanwhile, heat a non-stick frying pan over a medium heat. Toss in the sunflower seeds, drizzle the agave or honey over them, and add a pinch of salt. Cook, stirring frequently, until the syrup coats the seeds and they turn golden, about 3–4 minutes. (The seeds tend to stick to your stirring implement, so use a small spoon to scrape them back into the pan from time to time.) Remove the seeds to a plate to cool.

3 | Break the broccoli into pieces. Place in a food processor and whizz until very finely chopped. (Alternatively, grate the broccoli on the coarse side of a grater into a bowl.)

4 | Scrape the broccoli into a mixing bowl. Stir in the lemon juice and oil, and season well with salt and pepper. Peel the eggs and chop coarsely, then add to the broccoli and stir. Divide between two plates.

5 | Break up the seeds into small clusters, scatter over the salad, and serve. (If saving the second portion, keep the remaining seeds separate.)

\\ Keep in an airtight container in the fridge for up to 2 days. Keep the seed clusters separate in an airtight bag and combine with the salad just before serving.

MISO AUBERGINE & TOFU WITH RED CABBAGE SALAD

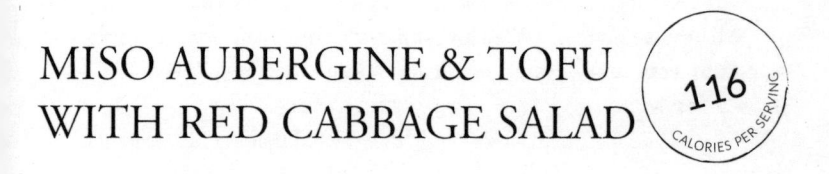

116 CALORIES PER SERVING

Gluten-free (if gluten-free miso and soy sauce are used) \\ Dairy-free \\ Vegan
NUTRITIONAL INFO PER SERVING: 4g fat, of which 0.4g saturates
13g carbohydrate, of which 8g sugars \\ 8g protein \\ 1.9g salt \\ 5g fibre

Aubergines, being full of water and sponge-like, cook brilliantly in the microwave and absorb flavours like a champ. Here they team up with nutritious tofu in a sweet miso and mirin dressing, on a bed of sharp, citrus-soaked red cabbage.

PREP & COOK TIME: **20 MINUTES, PLUS
10 MINUTES STANDING TIME**
SERVINGS: **2 LARGE**

150g/5½oz red cabbage
2 tbsp fresh lemon or lime juice
sea salt
200g/7oz/1 small–medium aubergine
  (eggplant)

100g/3½oz fresh firm tofu
1 spring onion (scallion)
2 tbsp miso
1 tbsp mirin
1 tsp dark soy sauce
½ tsp chilli flakes, or to taste
fresh coriander (cilantro), to garnish
  (optional)

1 Shred the cabbage as finely as possible and place in a bowl. Add the lemon or lime juice and a good pinch of salt, and stir. Set aside, stirring from time to time.

2 Cut the aubergine into 1cm/½in cubes and place in a microwave-safe container. Season lightly with salt and toss with your fingertips. Microwave on high power for 3 minutes, then stand for 2 minutes, until tender throughout. Strain and remove to a bowl to cool.

3 Meanwhile, pat the tofu dry and cut into 1cm/½in cubes. Slice the spring onion.

4 In a small bowl, beat together the miso, mirin and soy sauce until smooth. Stir in the chilli flakes.

5 Add the tofu, spring onion and miso dressing to the aubergine and stir to combine.

6 Leave everything to stand for 10–15 minutes and serve, or chill if you have time. Garnish with a handful of chopped coriander if you have it.

\\ Keep the cabbage and the aubergine mixture in separate airtight containers in the fridge for up to 3 days. Not suitable for freezing.

\\ Feed the non-fasters: Serve with cold egg noodles or soba noodles dressed with sesame oil.

SPICED GAZPACHO WITH LEMONY EGG

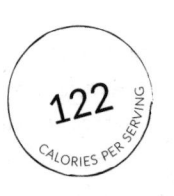

122 CALORIES PER SERVING

Gluten-free \\ Dairy-free \\ Vegan (if the egg is replaced with chickpeas)
NUTRITIONAL INFO PER SERVING: 6g fat, of which 2g saturates
9g carbohydrate, of which 9g sugars \\ 9g protein \\ 1g salt \\ 3g fibre

This refreshing 'liquid salad' is perfect on a warm day. I've spiced it up with toasted cumin and chilli, but leave these out if you prefer a classic gazpacho. The lemony egg topping is optional, but it does make it a complete meal, being filling and full of protein. Without it, the gazpacho has just 57 calories per serving. Alternatively (or in addition), scatter a chunk of crumbled feta on top (90 cals for 50g of reduced-fat feta or 127 cals for regular feta) or 60g/2¼oz/⅓ cup drained canned chickpeas (82 cals).

PREP & COOK TIME: **20 MINUTES**
SERVINGS: **2 LARGE**

2 eggs
½ tsp cumin seeds
100g/3½oz cucumber (about ⅓)
50g/1¾oz celery (1 large stick)
50g/1¾oz red pepper (about ½)
100g/3½oz tomatoes
25g/1oz red or regular onion (½ small)
1 garlic clove

250ml/9fl oz/generous 1 cup tomato juice
1 tsp best white or red wine vinegar, or to taste
sea salt and freshly ground black pepper
cayenne pepper or chilli flakes, to taste
ice cubes
squeeze of fresh lemon juice

1 Place the eggs in a small pan and cover with cold water. Bring to the boil, then reduce the heat and simmer for 10 minutes. Drain and cool under cold running water. Set aside.

2 | Heat a frying pan over a high heat and toss in the cumin seeds. Shake the pan and toast the seeds until they turn a shade darker and there is a whiff of cumin scent, about 1 minute, then remove the seeds to a plate to cool.

3 | Coarsely chop the cucumber, celery, red pepper, tomatoes and onion, and place in a blender. Crush in the garlic and add the tomato juice, vinegar, seasoning, chilli, and cumin seeds.

4 | Whizz the mixture on high speed for a short time until just combined but not utterly smooth, if you like a few chunks. Taste for seasoning.

5 | Pour the gazpacho into one or two bowls, add plenty of ice cubes and stir. Leave for about 5 minutes, then remove the ice. (Alternatively, chill the gazpacho for 2 or more hours until nice and cold.)

6 | Meanwhile, peel one or two of the eggs and mash in a bowl with a little salt, pepper and lemon juice.

7 | Serve the cold gazpacho with lemony egg on top.

\\ Freely add chopped fresh herbs to the bowl: dill, coriander, parsley, or basil (calories negligible).

\\ Can be served with half a pitta bread (62 cals), cold, toasted, or cut into strips and cooked in the oven until crunchy.

\\ Keep in an airtight container in the fridge for up to 3 days and serve straight from the fridge. Chill the second boiled egg in its shell; mash with the seasoning and lemon juice just before serving. Not suitable for freezing.

\\ Feed the non-fasters: Multiply ingredients as necessary and serve with tortilla chips topped with melted cheese, crusty bread, or a hot garlic baguette.

COLD CUCUMBER SOUP WITH WALNUTS

187
CALORIES PER SERVING

Gluten-free

NUTRITIONAL INFO PER SERVING: 12g fat, of which 2g saturates
11g carbohydrate, of which 11g sugars \\ 9g protein \\ 0.2g salt \\ 2g fibre

As long as your cucumber and yogurt are already well chilled, this won't require much extra chilling time. Crushed walnuts sprinkled on each bowl add texture, substance and protein to this Balkan-style summer soup.

PREP & COOK TIME: **10 MINUTES, PLUS 10 MINUTES OR MORE CHILLING TIME (OPTIONAL)**

SERVINGS: **2 LARGE**

250g/9oz (1 medium) cucumber, with skin
1 garlic clove

125ml/4fl oz/½ cup water
250g/9oz/1 cup low-fat yogurt
1 tsp white wine vinegar
large handful of fresh mint leaves
sea salt and freshly ground black pepper
25g/1oz walnuts

1 Cut the cucumber into large chunks.

2 Peel the garlic and remove any sprout. Place in the blender and whizz at high speed until chopped.

3 Add the cucumber, water, yogurt, vinegar and mint, and season well with salt and pepper. Whizz at high speed until relatively smooth. Taste for seasoning.

4 If you have time, chill for 10 minutes or more.

5   Chop or crush the walnuts, then sprinkle on top of each bowl of soup and serve.

\\ Chopped hard-boiled egg goes well with this as a topping if you need extra protein (72 cals per egg).

\\ Keep in an airtight container in the fridge for up to 3 days. Sprinkle with walnuts just before serving. Not suitable for freezing.

\\ Feed the non-fasters: Multiply ingredients as necessary and serve with toasted pitta bread or hot garlic bread.

MINTED CHICKPEA SOUP

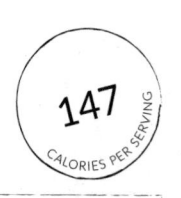

147 CALORIES PER SERVING

Gluten-free \\ Dairy-free \\ Vegan

NUTRITIONAL INFO PER SERVING: 4g fat, of which 0.5g saturates
19g carbohydrate, of which 1g sugars \\ 10g protein \\ 1.9g salt \\ 7g fibre

A whizz-bang bone-clinging bean soup. I discovered by accident that the dried mint in herbal teabags, usually a high-quality peppermint, is far superior to the usual stuff sold as a cooking herb, and tends to be fresher, so just snip open a couple of teabags for this recipe.

PREP & COOK TIME: **20 MINUTES**
SERVINGS: **2 MEDIUM**

1 garlic clove, peeled
225g/8oz/scant 1½ cups canned
  chickpeas (1 x 400g can, drained)

250ml/9fl oz/generous 1 cup water
1 tsp stock powder
1 lemon
2 tsp dried mint (see intro)
sea salt and freshly ground
  black pepper

1 Put the garlic in the blender and whizz at high speed until chopped. Add everything else and whizz at high speed until completely smooth.

2 Pour into a small saucepan and bring to the boil, then reduce the heat, simmer for 10 minutes, stirring occasionally, and serve.

\\ For a creamy tang, top with a heaped tablespoon of low-fat yogurt (27 cals).

\\ Feel free to add 50–100g/1¾–3½oz fresh steamed vegetables such as broccoli, courgette, spinach or chard (20–30 cals) to the finished soup. Alternatively, stir a large handful of baby spinach leaves into the soup at the end and stir until wilted (11 cals for 50g).

\\ Keep in an airtight container in the fridge for up to 3 days. Can also be frozen.

GREEK-STYLE EGG & LEMON SOUP WITH SAFFRON

144 CALORIES PER SERVING

Gluten-free \\ Dairy-free
NUTRITIONAL INFO PER SERVING: 4g fat, of which 1g saturates
8g carbohydrate, of which 4g sugars \\ 10g protein \\ 2.5g salt \\ 7g fibre

Traditional Greek avgolemono soup has a chicken and rice or pasta base, thickened and enriched with an emulsion of egg and lemon juice. My version is a quick and flavourful broth of leeks, cauliflower and courgette, with broad beans for extra protein. I've sexed it up with a little saffron, making it less pale and more interesting, but you could omit it.

PREP & COOK TIME: **20 MINUTES**
SERVINGS: **2 LARGE**

500ml/18fl oz/2 cups soup stock or 500ml/18fl oz/2 cups water + 2 tsp stock powder
100g/3½oz leek
100g/3½oz courgette (zucchini)
100g/3½oz cauliflower
100g/3½oz/⅔ cup broad (fava) beans, fresh or frozen

1 egg
1 tbsp fresh lemon juice, plus extra to serve
large pinch of saffron strands
sea salt and freshly ground black pepper
fresh chopped parsley, to serve (optional)

1   Put the stock or water in a saucepan and bring to the boil. (If using stock powder, stir it in to dissolve.)

2   Meanwhile, roughly chop the leek and courgette, and break the cauliflower into small florets.

3   Once the stock is boiling, add the leek, courgette and cauliflower, return to the boil, and simmer for 3 minutes.

4   Add the broad beans, return to the boil, and simmer for 3 minutes.

5   Meanwhile, in a medium bowl, combine the egg and lemon juice and whisk until frothy. Place the bowl near the cooker for the next step.

6   Add the saffron to the soup, stir and remove from the heat. Grab a ladle, a ½ cup measure or a teacup. Tilt the pan and remove a ladleful of liquid. While gently whisking the egg mixture, slowly pour in the liquid. Once incorporated, it should feel hot.

7   Still off the heat, stir the soup and gradually pour the egg mixture back into the pan. Keep stirring while the soup turns opaque and silky, about 2 minutes. Cover and stand for 2–3 minutes.

8   Stir well again and taste for seasoning, adding salt if necessary and a little more lemon, if desired. Top each bowl with parsley and black pepper.

\\ Keep in an airtight container in the fridge for up to 3 days; reheat thoroughly but do not boil to avoid curdling. Can also be frozen – thaw before reheating.

\\ Feed the non-fasters: Multiply ingredients as necessary and serve with crusty bread and butter.

BUTTERBEAN & ROSEMARY SOUP

101 CALORIES PER SERVING

Gluten-free \\ Dairy-free \\ Vegan

NUTRITIONAL INFO PER SERVING: 0.8g fat, of which 0.2g saturates
16g carbohydrate, of which 2g sugars \\ 8g protein \\ 2.g salt \\ 8g fibre

---

This remarkably simple, filling and creamy potage is done in a flash.

PREP & COOK TIME: **20 MINUTES**
SERVINGS: **2 MEDIUM**

2 x 5cm/2in sprigs of fresh rosemary
1 x 400g can butterbeans, drained
and rinsed

250ml/9fl oz/generous 1 cup soup
stock, or 250ml/9fl oz/generous
1 cup water + 1 tsp stock powder
1½ tbsp fresh lemon juice
sea salt and freshly ground
black pepper

1 Strip the rosemary leaves from the stem. Ideally, pound them briefly in a mortar to release the flavour.

2 Place the rosemary in the blender along with everything else and whizz at high speed until completely smooth – a good 3 minutes or so.

3 Pour into a small saucepan and bring to the boil, then reduce the heat, simmer for 10 minutes, stirring occasionally, and serve.

\\ For a creamy tang, top with a heaped tablespoon of low-fat yogurt (27 cals).

\\ Add a little extra flavour and nutrition by sprinkling with toasted sesame seeds (52 cals per tbsp).

\\ Top freely with fresh chopped parsley or chives (calories negligible).

\\ Feel free to add 50–100g/1¾–3½oz fresh steamed vegetables such as broccoli, courgette, spinach or chard (20–30 cals) to the finished soup. Alternatively, stir a large handful of baby spinach leaves into the soup at the end and stir until wilted (11 cals for 50g).

\\ Keep in an airtight container in the fridge for up to 3 days. Can also be frozen.

SPICY EGYPTIAN BEAN SOUP

127 CALORIES PER SERVING

Gluten-free \\ Dairy-free \\ Vegan
NUTRITIONAL INFO PER SERVING: 0.8g fat, of which 0.1g saturates
20g carbohydrate, of which 6g sugars \\ 10g protein \\ 1.2g salt \\ 8g fibre

The *ful medames* used here are dried broad beans or fava beans, which have been cooked and canned. They are enjoyed for breakfast in Egypt with garlic, lemon and hard-boiled eggs. Here they make a filling, velvety, protein-rich, super-quick soup. They can be found in Asian and Mediterranean markets.

PREP & COOK TIME: **20 MINUTES**
SERVINGS: **2 MEDIUM**

1 garlic clove, peeled
1 x 400g can *ful medames*, borlotti
  beans, pinto beans, or black beans,
  drained and rinsed
250ml/9fl oz/generous 1 cup soup
  stock, or 250ml/9fl oz/generous
  1 cup water + 1 tsp stock powder

1 tbsp fresh lemon juice
2 tsp honey or agave nectar
½ tsp cumin seeds or ground cumin
½ tsp paprika
¼ tsp chilli flakes, or to taste
sea salt and freshly ground
  black pepper

1. Put the garlic in the blender and whizz at high speed until chopped. Add everything else and whizz at high speed until completely smooth.

2. Pour into a small saucepan and bring to the boil, then reduce the heat, simmer for 10 minutes, stirring occasionally, and serve.

\\ For a creamy tang, top with a heaped tablespoon of low-fat yogurt (27 cals).

\\ Feel free to add 50–100g/1¾–3½oz fresh steamed vegetables such as broccoli, courgette, spinach or chard (20–30 cals) to the finished soup. Alternatively, stir a large handful of baby spinach leaves into the soup at the end and stir until wilted (11 cals for 50g).

\\ Keep in an airtight container in the fridge for up to 3 days. Can also be frozen.

NEON RED PEPPER SOUP

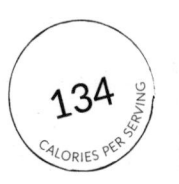

134 CALORIES PER SERVING

Gluten-free \\ Dairy-free \\ Vegan
NUTRITIONAL INFO PER SERVING: 2g fat, of which 0.4g saturates
26g carbohydrate, of which 25g sugars \\ 5g protein \\ trace salt \\ 9g fibre

You'll soon see how this lightning-quick soup got its name! Its flavour and texture match its gorgeous appearance. The quality and ripeness of the peppers will vary the intensity of the soup's colour and sweetness, but it never fails to deliver a dazzling orange hue. Although roasting peppers brings out the best flavour, cooking them in the microwave is quick and renders the skins soft enough to purée, so no fiddly peeling, and still intensifies the flavour. Alternatively, you could boil or steam them for 8–10 minutes until thoroughly soft.

PREP & COOK TIME: **20 MINUTES**
SERVINGS: **2 LARGE**

800g/1lb 12oz (about 4) red peppers

sea salt
2 garlic cloves
1 small fresh red or green chilli
2 tbsp fresh lemon juice

1. Core and deseed the peppers and cut into chunks. Place in a large microwave-safe dish and sprinkle with salt (no need to add water). Cover and microwave on high power for 7 minutes (the peppers should be tender throughout when prodded with a knife), then stand for 2 minutes. Remove the lid and leave to cool briefly.

2. Meanwhile, peel the garlic and remove any sprout. Place the garlic in the blender and whizz at high speed until chopped. Using scissors, snip the chilli into the blender.

3. Once the peppers are cooled, add them to the blender, along with any cooking juices.

4. Add the lemon juice. Whizz at high speed until thoroughly blended.

5. Taste for seasoning, adding more salt if necessary.

6. Eat while still warm. Alternatively, reheat in a saucepan until just below boiling. Can also be enjoyed chilled.

\\ Enjoy on its own or with half a pitta bread (62 cals). Top freely with chopped fresh coriander, parsley or chives (calories negligible). If serving cold, garnish with chopped cucumber.

\\ For a creamy tang, top with a heaped tablespoon of low-fat yogurt (27 cals). For extra protein, top with chopped hard-boiled egg (72 cals per egg).

\\ Keep in an airtight container in the fridge for up to 3 days. Can also be frozen.

\\ Feed the non-fasters: Accompany with crusty bread and top with crème fraîche and toasted flaked almonds.

PAPPA AL POMODORO

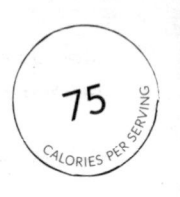

75 CALORIES PER SERVING

Dairy-free \\ Vegan
NUTRITIONAL INFO PER SERVING: 0.6g fat, of which 0.1g saturates
14g carbohydrate, of which 6g sugars \\ 4g protein \\ 1.6g salt \\ 2g fibre

Though not massively high in protein, this classic Italian peasant-style dish is filling and delectable, as a naughty bit of crusty bread soaks up a juicy, sweet tomato soup. This could also be made with 400g/14oz fresh cherry tomatoes in place of canned – crush them slightly with a potato masher once cooked.

PREP & COOK TIME: **20 MINUTES**
SERVINGS: **2 LARGE**

1 x 400g can cherry tomatoes or
  chopped tomatoes
½ tsp finest balsamic vinegar
1 tsp stock powder
100ml/3½fl oz water

2 garlic cloves, crushed
large pinch of dried mixed herbs
sea salt and freshly ground
  black pepper
¼ tsp agave nectar or honey (optional)
handful of fresh basil leaves
25g/1oz piece sourdough or country
  bread, lightly toasted

1   Put the tomatoes, balsamic, stock powder, water, garlic and dried herbs in a saucepan, and season with salt and pepper. Stir and bring to the boil over a high heat, then reduce the heat and simmer for 10 minutes, stirring occasionally. Remove from the heat.

2   Taste for seasoning: add agave or honey if desired (this will depend on the natural sweetness of the tomatoes).

3   Tear the basil leaves into the soup, then the bread, tearing it into bite-sized chunks. (Note: If saving the second portion, don't add the bread

now: add it when the soup is reheated.) Stir well, cover and set aside for 5 minutes for the flavours to get acquainted and the bread to soften.

4 Serve in soup bowls with more black pepper and torn basil, if desired.

\\ At just 75 cals per serving, you can probably afford to finish each bowl with a delicious, measured splash of extra-virgin olive oil (40 cals per tsp).

\\ Keep the tomato soup, without the bread, in an airtight container in the fridge for up to 3 days. Can also be frozen. Reheat and add the bread as in step 3.

\\ Feed the non-fasters: Drizzle the finished bowls with extra-virgin olive oil and Parmesan shavings.

MISO NOODLE BOWL

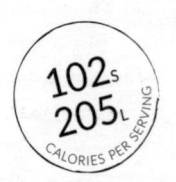

102 s
205 L
CALORIES PER SERVING

Gluten-free (if gluten-free miso and noodles are used) \\ Dairy-free \\ Vegan
NUTRITIONAL INFO PER SERVING: (1 large serving) 8g fat, of which 0.7g saturates
15g carbohydrate, of which 2g sugars \\ 17g protein \\ 3g salt \\ 4g fibre

This is my favourite fast-day meal for one: it's super-filling, quick, yummy and maxed-out on health bonuses. It's quite substantial and sometimes I can't finish it, so I'll cool and refrigerate it to polish off later, reheated in the microwave with some extra steamed veggies, perhaps adding a sliced spring onion, some chopped fresh coriander, or a handful of sprouts for variety.

Low-fat ramen noodles (38 cals for half a packet) are a quick addition here, but by all means use shirataki noodles, cooking them according to the instructions on page 116, and you can subtract calories! Or use your favourite quick-cooking noodles and substitute their calorie count for the 38 cals.

PREP & COOK TIME: **20 MINUTES**
SERVINGS: **1 LARGE OR 2 SMALL**

1 garlic clove or ½ tsp garlic powder
  or granules
1cm/½in piece fresh ginger
1 red chilli or 2 tsp chilli sauce, or
  to taste
100g/3½oz fresh firm tofu

100g/3½oz mixed fresh broccoli and
  cabbage or kale
25g/1oz/about 1 heaped tbsp miso
  paste
1 tsp stock powder (optional)
½ packet (approx. 40g) dried low-fat
  ramen noodles
squeeze of fresh lime or lemon juice

1. Boil a small amount of water in the kettle. Meanwhile, crush the garlic, peel and grate the ginger, slice the chilli (if using), cut the tofu into cubes, cut the broccoli into small florets, and shred the cabbage or kale.

2. Once boiled, leave the water to settle and cool for a minute or two.

3. Measure the miso into a cup or small bowl. Pour a splash of hot water over it and stir to dissolve the miso. (Using hot, not boiling, water maintains the optimum nutrition in the miso and prevents it from curdling.)

4. Pour about 200–250ml of the boiled water into a small saucepan. Add a little stock powder if desired, the garlic, ginger and chilli. Stir and bring to the boil.

5. Add the noodles, tofu and vegetables and bring to the boil, then cook, stirring frequently, just until the noodles are soft and the veg are barely tender, about 2 minutes.

6. Remove from the heat, cover and allow to stand for 1 minute, then stir in the dissolved miso. Add a squeeze of lime and eat immediately.

\\ Feel free to top with chopped or sliced spring onions, a handful of chopped fresh coriander, bean sprouts or salad sprouts (calories negligible).

\\ Best eaten immediately or on the same day. Not suitable for freezing.

CLASSIC STIR-FRY WITH TOFU

134 CALORIES PER SERVING

Gluten-free (if gluten-free soy sauce is used) \\ Dairy-free \\ Vegan

NUTRITIONAL INFO PER SERVING: 5g fat, of which 0.6g saturates

15g carbohydrate, of which 11g sugars \\ 8g protein \\ 3g salt \\ 4g fibre

A stir-fry is an instinctual go-to meal for using up lots of veggies, and here's a winning formula for fast days. Use what vegetables you have to hand, weighing a total of 300g. My typical combo is used below. You could also use mangetout, bean sprouts, and/or water chestnuts. I always use mirin but you could substitute another cooking wine (see page 36).

PREP & COOK TIME: **20 MINUTES**
SERVINGS: **2 MEDIUM**

300g/10½oz mixed veg: ½ red pepper,
  broccoli, cauliflower, Savoy cabbage,
  courgette (zucchini)
100g/3½oz fresh firm tofu
1 small red onion (about 25g/1oz)

2 tbsp dark soy sauce
1 tbsp mirin
1 tsp cornflour (cornstarch)
1 tsp sunflower oil
pinch of salt
pinch of sugar
1 small hot chilli
squeeze of fresh lime (optional)

1 Cut the pepper into strips and the rest of the veg into bite-sized pieces.

2 Pat the tofu dry and cut into 1cm/½in cubes. Slice the onion.

3 In a small bowl or cup, mix together the soy sauce, mirin and cornflour.

4 Heat a large non-stick lidded frying pan or wok over a high heat until very hot.

5 | Add the oil, tofu and onion and a pinch of salt and sugar, and stir. Using scissors, snip the chilli into the pan. Stir frequently until the onion is soft and the tofu is patched with brown, about 3 minutes. Remove the contents of the pan to a plate and return the pan to the heat.

6 | Chuck in the veg and 1 tbsp water, and stir. Cover to allow the veg to steam, stirring occasionally, until the veg have just started to soften, about 2 minutes.

7 | Add the sauce mixture and stir – it should start to thicken immediately. Add the tofu mixture and stir through the sauce until evenly mixed and hot throughout. Serve immediately, with a squeeze of lime if desired.

\\ Feel free to top with chopped or sliced spring onions, a handful of chopped fresh coriander or salad sprouts (calories negligible).

\\ Enjoy on its own, or serve on top of ½ cup cooked brown rice (108 cals), or with cooked shirataki noodles (calories negligible; page 116).

\\ Best eaten immediately or on the same day. Not suitable for freezing.

SPANISH STIR-FRY WITH CUMIN-YOGURT SAUCE

137 CALORIES PER SERVING

Gluten-free

NUTRITIONAL INFO PER SERVING: 5g fat, of which 0.8g saturates
15g carbohydrate, of which 6g sugars \\ 9g protein \\ 0.5g salt \\ 6g fibre

This simple Cumin-Yogurt sauce outdoes itself in the deliciousness stakes, and I've also used it as an optional addition to Mango & Black Bean Salad (page 51). Try it also with potatoes, boiled eggs and as a salad dressing.

PREP & COOK TIME: **20 MINUTES**
SERVINGS: **2 MEDIUM**

50g/1¾oz cabbage greens such as kale, cavolo nero or Savoy cabbage, torn from stems (prepared weight)
150g/5½oz mushrooms
1 tsp extra-virgin rapeseed or olive oil
sea salt and ground black pepper
1 garlic clove

100g/3½oz cherry tomatoes
125g/4½oz/¾ cup canned chickpeas (½ x 400g can, drained)
1 tsp smoked paprika (pimentón), mild or hot

Cumin-Yogurt Sauce

100g/3½oz low-fat yogurt
½ tsp ground cumin
2 tsp fresh lemon juice

1. Roughly chop the cabbage and tear or thickly slice the mushrooms.

2. Heat a large lidded frying pan over a medium–high heat. Add the oil, cabbage and mushrooms with a pinch of salt and stir. Add 2 tbsp water and stir again. Cover the pan and cook, stirring occasionally, until the mushrooms are juicy and the cabbage has collapsed, about 3 minutes. Meanwhile, crush the garlic and halve the tomatoes.

3. Add the garlic, tomatoes, chickpeas and smoked paprika to the pan. Cook, stirring, until the tomatoes soften slightly. Grind in some pepper, stir, cover and set aside.

4. To make the sauce, measure the yogurt into a small bowl, beat in the cumin and lemon juice, and season well with salt and pepper. Serve spooned over the stir-fry.

\\ Enjoy on its own or with a serving of Cauliflower Couscous (page 118; 42 cals), ½ cup cooked brown rice (108 cals), or half a pitta bread (62 cals). Also lovely served on a bed of steamed spinach (25 cals per 100g raw spinach).

\\ Top freely with fresh chopped parsley (calories negligible).

\\ Keep in an airtight container in the fridge for up to 3 days, keeping the sauce separate. The stir-fry can be frozen, but make the sauce fresh before serving.

\\ Feed the non-fasters: Accompany with rice, couscous, or crusty bread.

TOPPED FLATBREADS

This easy fast-day treat is a canvas for your imagination. You can eat them like mini pizzas or roll up or fold into a hot sandwich. The total calories involved depend mainly on your flatbread, which could be a wrap, tortilla, Arabic khobez, part of a lavash, or even a pitta bread slashed open and opened flat. Flatbreads of all kinds freeze well if frozen fresh, and they thaw quickly, so keep some handy for fast days, ready to pile with toppings. Here are two winning combos, which, if you use a flatbread under 150 cals, will clock you in around the 300-cal mark for a generous serving. The recipes serve one and are easily doubled or multiplied as necessary to feed more.

THREE-TOMATO & MOZZARELLA FLATBREAD

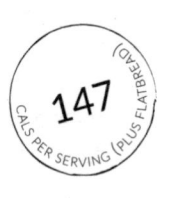

147 CALS PER SERVING (PLUS FLATBREAD)

NUTRITIONAL INFO PER SERVING: 6g fat, of which 4g saturates

0g carbohydrate, of which 3g sugars \\ 14g protein \\ 1.6g salt \\ 4g fibre

---

PREP & COOK TIME: **26–28 MINUTES**
SERVINGS: **1 LARGE**

3 sun-dried tomatoes (not in oil)
60g/2¼oz (½ a ball) half-fat mozzarella
3 cherry tomatoes

1 flatbread (see intro)
1 tsp tomato purée (paste)
a sprinkle of garlic powder or granules
3 basil tips or 10 leaves
sea salt and freshly ground
   black pepper

1   Preheat the oven to 200°C/400°F/Gas Mark 6.

2   Boil the kettle. Put the sun-dried tomatoes in a small bowl and pour boiling water over them to cover. Set aside for 15 minutes to soften.

3   Meanwhile, thinly slice the mozzarella and slice the cherry tomatoes.

4   Line a baking sheet with non-stick baking parchment and place the flatbread on it. Spread the tomato purée over the bread and sprinkle lightly with garlic powder.

5   Squeeze and pat dry the sun-dried tomatoes and chop coarsely, then scatter over the flatbread. Add the mozzarella and cherry tomatoes, tear over the basil, and season with salt and pepper.

6   Bake for 6–8 minutes, until the cheese is melted and the flatbread is crisped to your liking, then serve. (If rolling or folding for a hot sandwich, you may prefer it less crisp.)

\\ Best eaten fresh. Keep leftovers in an airtight container in the fridge for up to 24 hours, then reheat in the oven. Not suitable for freezing.

\\ Feed the non-fasters: Multiply ingredients as necessary and add mozzarella or grated pizza cheese and a drizzle of olive oil before baking.

SPICY MEXICAN BEAN FLATBREAD

150 CALS PER SERVING (PLUS FLATBREAD)

NUTRITIONAL INFO PER SERVING: 4g fat, of which 2g saturates
19g carbohydrate, of which 3g sugars \\ 10g protein \\ 2.1g salt \\ 8g fibre

PREP & COOK TIME: **11–13 MINUTES**
SERVINGS: **1 LARGE**

1 flatbread (see intro)
100g/3½oz canned refried beans

1 spring onion (scallion)
3 cherry tomatoes
1 tsp capers in vinegar, drained
2 tsp jalapeños in vinegar, drained
10g/¼oz Parmesan cheese, grated

1 Preheat the oven to 200°C/400°F/Gas Mark 6.

2 Line a baking sheet with non-stick baking parchment and place the flatbread on it. Spread the refried beans over the bread.

3 Slice the spring onion and cherry tomatoes and scatter over the beans, adding the capers and jalapeños. Sprinkle the Parmesan over everything.

4 Bake for 6–8 minutes, until the surface is bubbling and the flatbread is crisped to your liking, then serve. (If rolling or folding for a hot sandwich, you may prefer it less crisp.)

\\ Serve with a low-cal Mexican salsa.

\\ Best eaten fresh. Keep leftovers in an airtight container in the fridge for up to 24 hours, then reheat in the oven. Not suitable for freezing.

\\ Feed the non-fasters: Multiply ingredients as necessary and add grated Cheddar or pizza cheese and a drizzle of olive oil before baking.

CHEESY COURGETTE & DILL PANCAKES

141 CALORIES PER SERVING

NUTRITIONAL INFO PER SERVING: 7g fat, of which 2g saturates
9g carbohydrate, of which 3g sugars \\ 12g protein \\ 0.6g salt \\ 1g fibre

Grated courgette forms the low-cal bulk of these Greek-style fritters. Cottage cheese works beautifully in savoury or sweet pancakes, adding tang and substance but few calories. Use 1 tsp dried dill if fresh isn't available.

PREP & COOK TIME: **25 MINUTES**
SERVINGS: **2 MEDIUM**

100g/3½oz/½ cup cottage cheese
150g/5½oz/1 medium courgette
  (zucchini)
sea salt

handful of fresh dill
1 spring onion (scallion)
1 garlic clove
1 tbsp plain flour
¼ tsp baking powder
1 egg
1 tsp olive oil

1 Measure the cottage cheese and place in a sieve over the sink to drain.

2 Coarsely grate the courgette into a bowl. Sprinkle generously with salt and mix thoroughly with your hands. Set aside for 10 minutes while you prepare the rest of the ingredients.

3 Chop the dill, slice the spring onion, crush the garlic; place them in a bowl with the flour, baking powder and egg. Beat thoroughly.

4 Squeeze handfuls of courgette to remove excess liquid, then add to the egg mixture.

5 Add the drained cottage cheese to the egg mixture and beat well.

6 Place a non-stick frying pan over a medium heat. Add the olive oil to the pan. Using a dessertspoon, scoop spoonfuls of the courgette batter into the oil and gently press the top to form pancakes roughly 7cm/3in in diameter. (You may only be able to fit four at a time in the pan; you could keep the first batch warm in the oven while you cook the rest.)

7 Cook until the underside is dark golden. Flip over and cook the other side until done, then serve hot.

\\ Accompany with steamed veggies dressed with fresh lemon juice, or a tomato and onion salad on a bed of spinach dressed with balsamic vinegar.

\\ Keep, covered on a plate, in the fridge for up to 3 days. Reheat on a baking sheet in a 200°C/400°F/Gas Mark 6 oven for about 5–7 minutes, until you can hear them sizzling when you listen closely. Can also be frozen; reheat from frozen for about 10 minutes.

\\ Feed the non-fasters: Multiply ingredients as necessary and serve with the accompaniments suggested above, adding olive oil and Parmesan shavings.

COURGETTE & FETA FRITTATA

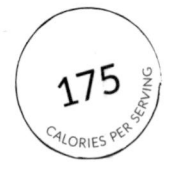
175 CALORIES PER SERVING

Gluten-free

NUTRITIONAL INFO PER SERVING: 12g fat, of which 4g saturates
3g carbohydrate, of which 3g sugars \\ 14g protein \\ 0.8g salt \\ 2g fibre

Here's one of my all-time favourite uses for courgettes, reworked for 5:2. The courgettes may seem to crowd the pan at first, but don't worry – they shrink considerably as they turn golden. If reduced-fat feta isn't available, use ordinary feta and add 19 cals per serving. Enjoy this hot, warm or cold and at any time of day.

PREP & COOK TIME: **20 MINUTES**
SERVINGS: **2 LARGE**

300g/10½oz/about 2 medium
  courgettes (zucchini)

2 tsp extra-virgin rapeseed oil or
  olive oil
sea salt and freshly ground
  black pepper
2 eggs
50g/1¾oz reduced-fat feta cheese

1. Slice the courgettes quite thinly: about 3mm/⅛in.

2. Heat a grillproof non-stick frying pan over a medium–high heat and add the oil and the courgettes, season with salt and pepper, and stir.

3. Cook, stirring frequently, until each piece is soft and tinged with gold, about 8–10 minutes.

4. Meanwhile, beat the eggs together with a fork until well combined.

5. Spread the courgettes evenly over the base of the pan. Pour in the eggs evenly over the courgettes.

6. Preheat the grill to high.

7. Crumble the feta over the egg mixture.

8. Cook until the underside is light golden, about 2 minutes, then place the pan under the grill until the top is set, about 1–2 minutes. Remove from pan, cut into 4 wedges and serve. Can also be eaten warm or cold.

\\ Top freely with chopped fresh dill or parsley, or some fresh thyme leaves (calories negligible).

\\ Keep in an airtight container in the fridge for up to 3 days. Not suitable for freezing.

\\ Feed the non-fasters: Serve with a tomato and onion salad with balsamic vinegar and olive oil, plus bread or potatoes.

CREAMY PAPRIKA MUSHROOMS

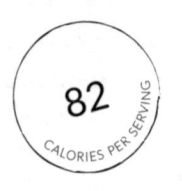

82 CALORIES PER SERVING

Gluten-free

NUTRITIONAL INFO PER SERVING: 3g fat, of which 0.7g saturates

10g carbohydrate, of which 5g sugars \\ 5g protein \\ 0.1g salt \\ 2g fibre

This Hungarian-style dish, singing with garlic and dill, suspends juicy mushrooms in a creamy, flavourful gravy, and marries perfectly with Cauliflower Couscous (page 118) or Shirataki Noodles (page 116). It works well with scrambled eggs, but can also be enjoyed on its own. Use ordinary mushrooms or a mixture of cultivated and wild. Be sure to use fresh, high-quality paprika and not a bottle of dust that has been languishing in the cupboard.

PREP & COOK TIME: **20 MINUTES**
SERVINGS: **2 MEDIUM**

3 spring onions (scallions)
1 tsp olive oil
200g/7oz mushrooms, regular or
  mixed wild and cultivated,
  brushed clean

sea salt and freshly ground
  black pepper
small handful of fresh dill
125g/4½oz/½ cup low-fat yogurt
2 tsp cornflour (cornstarch)
2 garlic cloves
2 tsp paprika
cayenne pepper, to finish (optional)

1. Chop the onions. Heat a large, lidded, non-stick frying pan over a medium heat and add the oil and the onions. Cook, stirring occasionally, until the onions are soft. Meanwhile, cut or tear the mushrooms into chunky pieces.

2 Add the mushrooms to the pan with salt, pepper, and 2 tbsp water. Cover and cook, stirring frequently, until the mushrooms are soft and juicy, about 3–4 minutes.

3 Meanwhile chop the dill – you should have about 2 rounded tbsp. Measure the yogurt into a small bowl and beat in the cornflour until smooth.

4 Reduce the heat and crush the garlic into the pan. Add the paprika and stir well.

5 Add 2 more tbsp water, then add the dill and stir well.

6 Turn the heat right down and stir in the yogurt mixture. Stir thoroughly until the sauce turns evenly reddish-brown and just starts to bubble, then remove from the heat. Eat immediately, sprinkled with cayenne if desired.

\\ This is just perfect with a portion of Cauliflower Couscous (page 118; 42 cals) to absorb all the creamy sauce. Alternatively, pair up with shirataki noodles (calories negligible) or low-fat noodles, ½ cup cooked brown rice (108 cals), or half a pitta bread (62 cals) or other bread. For extra protein, serve with a scrambled egg (72 cals).

\\ Keep in an airtight container in the fridge for up to 3 days. Can also be frozen. Reheat in the microwave: stir very thoroughly, as the sauce might curdle slightly at first, but stirring should emulsify it, and it is still delicious.

\\ Feed the non-fasters: Multiply ingredients as necessary and serve with spaghetti or pasta shapes and finish with a little crème fraîche and/or grated Parmesan cheese.

SWEET LENTIL CABBAGE WRAPS

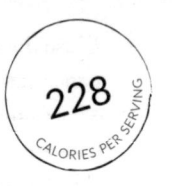

228 CALORIES PER SERVING

Gluten-free \\ Dairy-free \\ Vegan
NUTRITIONAL INFO PER SERVING: 3g fat, of which 0.4g saturates
37g carbohydrate, of which 10g sugars \\ 14g protein \\ 0.1g salt \\ 7g fibre

Here's an old favourite combo of mine reinvented for 5:2 to be low-cal and fuss-free – a deceptively humble-sounding yet remarkably delicious trio of lemony lentils, sweet caramelized onions and Savoy cabbage. Trust me, it's a winner.

PREP & COOK TIME: **30 MINUTES**
SERVINGS: **2 LARGE**

100g/3½oz red lentils
300ml/10fl oz/1¼ cups water
sea salt and freshly ground
  black pepper

200g/7oz/about 2 medium red onions
1 tsp olive oil
1 large unwaxed lemon
½ tsp agave nectar or honey
4 Savoy cabbage leaves

1. Rinse the lentils under cold water, then place in a small lidded pan and add the water. Bring to the boil and simmer, covered, for 15–20 minutes, stirring occasionally, until cooked to a porridge-like consistency. If the lentils seem too dry, add a splash more water. After about 10 minutes of cooking, season with salt.

2. Meanwhile, halve and slice the onions. Heat a lidded non-stick pan over a medium heat and add the oil. Add the onions and stir, then add 1 tbsp water and stir again. Cover and cook, stirring occasionally, until soft and caramelized, about 10 minutes.

3. Wash the lemon well and grate the zest, taking care not to remove any of the pith. Squeeze the juice.

4. When the lentils are cooked, stir in the lemon zest, 2 tbsp lemon juice, and the agave or honey. Stir in the onions, cover and set aside. (If saving the second portion, cool this mixture and reserve.)

5. Wash the cabbage leaves well and, retaining a bit of the washing water, place in a large microwave-safe container. Season each leaf lightly with salt. Cook on high power for 2 minutes, or until soft.

6. Place two cabbage leaves on each plate and spoon the lentil mixture over half, then fold over the leaves and serve.

\\ For a creamy tang, top with a heaped tablespoon of low-fat yogurt (27 cals).

\\ Keep the lentil mixture, covered, in the fridge for up to 3 days; cook the cabbage leaves just before serving. The mixture can also be frozen; reheat in the microwave.

\\ Feed the non-fasters: Multiply ingredients as necessary and serve with wholegrain rice. Top with crème fraîche.

EGGS POACHED IN RED PEPPER SAUCE

174 CALORIES PER SERVING

Gluten-free \\ Dairy-free

NUTRITIONAL INFO PER SERVING: 8g fat, of which 2g saturates

15g carbohydrate, of which 14g sugars \\ 10g protein \\ 0.4g salt \\ 4g fibre

---

Inspired by the Middle Eastern classic shakshouka, this dazzling dish is great for breakfast, lunch or dinner. Its delectable flavour profile is punctuated by cinnamon and dried mint – but don't rush out and buy a jar of dried mint: the best dried mint can be found in peppermint teabags, so just snip one open and use the pungent herb inside. This dish is actually improved by using very little oil because the peppers char in the pan and take on a gorgeous smoky flavour.

PREP & COOK TIME: **30 MINUTES**

SERVINGS: **2 LARGE**

1 small onion
1 red pepper
1 tsp olive oil
1 garlic clove
1 x 400g can chopped tomatoes

½ tsp balsamic or wine vinegar
½ tsp honey or agave nectar
½ tsp dried mint (see intro)
⅛ tsp ground cinnamon
large pinch of cayenne or chilli flakes
sea salt and freshly ground
  black pepper
2 eggs

1 Halve the onion and slice thinly. Core, deseed and thinly slice the red pepper.

2 Heat a large, lidded, non-stick frying pan over a medium–high heat. Add the olive oil, onion and red pepper. Cook, stirring frequently, for 5 minutes or until softened.

3 Crush the garlic into the pan and stir until fragrant, then add the remaining ingredients, except the eggs. Bring to the boil, then cover and simmer, stirring occasionally, for 10 minutes, until thickened.

4 (Note: If saving one portion for your next fast day, set aside half the sauce and cook just one egg now.) Use the back of a spoon to make two hollows in the sauce, then crack an egg into each one. Cover the pan and cook the eggs until done to the desired consistency, then serve.

\\ Can be served with Cauliflower Couscous (page 118; 42 cals), half a pitta bread (62 cals), ½ cup cooked brown rice (108 cals), or ½ cup cooked bulgur wheat (75 cals).

\\ Freely add chopped fresh herbs such as dill, parsley, mint or basil (calories negligible).

\\ If saving one portion for your next fast day, cook just one egg the first time, keep half the sauce in the fridge for up to 3 days or freeze it, then thaw, reheat and cook the egg in the sauce as above.

\\ Feed the non-fasters: Multiply ingredients as necessary, then top with crumbled feta or grated Cheddar, Gouda or Gruyère, or slices of fried halloumi cheese. Serve with crusty bread, wholegrain rice, couscous, or bulgur wheat.

GEORGIAN-STYLE BEANS IN WALNUT & CORIANDER SAUCE

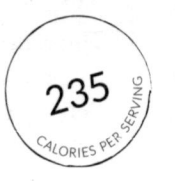

235 CALORIES PER SERVING

Gluten-free \\ Dairy-free \\ Vegan (excluding yogurt garnish)
NUTRITIONAL INFO PER SERVING: 11g fat, of which 1g saturates
23g carbohydrate, of which 7g sugars \\ 11g protein \\ 1.3g salt \\ 11g fibre

A creamy, spiced walnut sauce and kidney beans join forces to create a protein-packed dish that resembles a bean chilli when served warm, but can also be enjoyed cold on a heap of salad leaves. I've listed the optional garnishes below because they certainly make the dish prettier, but what the dish lacks in appearance, it more than makes up for with the rich, exotic flavour.

PREP & COOK TIME: **25 MINUTES**
SERVINGS: **2 LARGE**

1 garlic clove
2 spring onions (scallions)
25g/1oz/3 tbsp walnuts
handful of (about 15g/½ oz) fresh
    coriander (cilantro), roughly chopped
3–4 sprigs of fresh thyme, leaves
    stripped, or ½ tsp dried thyme
large pinch of ground cinnamon
large pinch of chilli flakes or
    cayenne pepper

1 tbsp balsamic vinegar
½ tsp agave nectar or honey
sea salt
6 tbsp water
1 tsp olive oil
1 x 400g can red kidney beans

Optional garnishes
chopped fresh coriander (cilantro)
fresh pomegranate seeds
    (15 cals per tbsp)
low-fat yogurt
    (27 cals per heaped tbsp)

1. Throw the garlic into the blender and whizz until chopped.

2. Roughly chop the spring onions and pop them in, along with the walnuts, coriander, thyme, cinnamon, chilli, balsamic vinegar, agave or honey, a good pinch of salt, and the water. Whizz at high speed until completely smooth.

3. Meanwhile, drain the beans.

4. Heat a small saucepan over a medium heat. Add the oil to the pan, then pour the contents of the blender into the pan, scraping out every last drop.

5. Simmer the sauce for about 3 minutes, stirring frequently, until slightly thickened.

6. Add the drained beans. Cook, stirring frequently, for 5 minutes.

7. Remove from the heat and leave to stand for 5 minutes, then serve, with garnishes if desired.

\\ Enjoy on its own or with Cauliflower Couscous (page 118; 42 cals), or some baby spinach leaves or steamed vegetables stirred through.

\\ Accompany with half a pitta bread (62 cals) or ½ cup cooked brown rice (108 cals).

\\ Keep, covered, in the fridge for up to 3 days. Reheat and serve hot or eat cold or at room temperature on a bed of salad leaves. Can also be frozen – thaw before reheating for best results.

\\ Feed the non-fasters: Multiply ingredients as necessary and serve with wholegrain rice and extra chopped walnuts scattered over.

GREEK-STYLE BUTTERBEANS WITH HERBS & TOMATOES

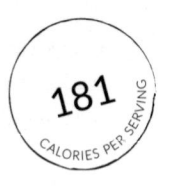

181 CALORIES PER SERVING

Gluten-free \\ Dairy-free \\ Vegan

NUTRITIONAL INFO PER SERVING: 3g fat, of which 0.4g saturates

30g carbohydrate, of which 15g sugars \\ 9g protein \\ 1.5g salt \\ 10g fibre

Creamy, filling butterbeans love the company of tomatoes and herbs, and it's the dill here that really works the magic.

PREP & COOK TIME: **20 MINUTES**

SERVINGS: **2 LARGE**

1 small onion or 3 spring onions
  (scallions)
1 tsp olive oil
2 garlic cloves
1 x 400g can butterbeans, drained
  and rinsed
1 x 400g can chopped tomatoes

sea salt and freshly ground
  black pepper
handful of fresh dill or 1 tsp dried dill
handful of fresh parsley
large sprig of fresh thyme or ½ tsp
  dried thyme
½ tsp dried oregano
2 tsp honey or agave nectar
2 tsp white or red wine vinegar

1   Chop the onions. Heat a non-stick frying pan over a medium–high heat and add the olive oil. Add the onion and cook, stirring frequently, until lightly golden and soft.

2   Crush the garlic into the pan and stir, then add the beans and tomatoes, season with salt and pepper, and stir. Reduce the heat to a medium simmer.

3   Chop the fresh herbs (if using) and add to the pan, along with the remaining ingredients. Cook, stirring occasionally, for about 10 more minutes, until most of the liquid has evaporated. Taste for seasoning and serve hot or at room temperature.

\\ Enjoy on its own or with Cauliflower Couscous (page 118; 42 cals), half a pitta bread (62 cals), or ½ cup cooked brown rice (108 cals). Delicious topped with a heaped tablespoon of low-fat yogurt (27 cals).

\\ Keep in an airtight container in the fridge for up to 3 days; the flavour really improves over time. Reheat in the microwave or serve at room temperature. Can also be frozen.

\\ Feed the non-fasters: Multiply ingredients as necessary and serve with wholegrain rice, couscous, crusty bread, or a garlic baguette.

VEGETABLE & CHICKPEA TAGINE

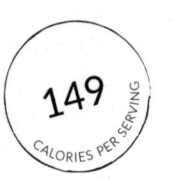

Gluten-free \\ Dairy-free \\ Vegan

NUTRITIONAL INFO PER SERVING: 3g fat, of which 0.4g saturates

23g carbohydrate, of which 13g sugars \\ 9g protein \\ 0.6g salt \\ 10g fibre

This super-flexible recipe is ridiculously easy and low in calories, yet staggeringly tempting, as your home fills with the exotic aromas of cinnamon and cumin.

PREP & COOK TIME: **25 MINUTES**

SERVINGS: **2 LARGE**

4 spring onions (scallions)

sea salt

100g/3½oz tomatoes

125g/4½oz/¾ cup canned chickpeas
   (½ x 400g can, drained)

1 tsp ground cumin

½ tsp ground cinnamon

¼ tsp chilli flakes, or to taste

2 tbsp tomato purée (paste)

1 tsp honey or agave nectar

½ tsp balsamic vinegar

Vegetable base

Choose a mix of any of the following,
   weighing 300g/10½oz:

butternut squash, peeled

carrot, peeled

cauliflower

courgette (zucchini)

celeriac, peeled

celery, stalks, heart and leaves

cucumber, seeds scraped out

daikon radish (mooli), peeled

fennel

peppers and fat chillies, deseeded

turnips, kohlrabi or swede (rutabaga),
   peeled

1　Cut the vegetables into chunks, and slice the spring onions.

2　Heat a saucepan over a medium–high heat and add the onions and veg, plus 2 tbsp water and a generous pinch of salt. Cover and steam for 3 minutes. Meanwhile, chop the tomato and assemble the remaining ingredients.

3　Once the veg have started to soften, add the remaining ingredients plus 125ml/4fl oz/½ cup water. Stir and bring to the boil, then reduce the heat to a simmer.

4　Cook for 10 minutes, stirring occasionally, until the veg have softened and the sauce has thickened. Serve.

\\ For a creamy tang, top with a heaped tablespoon of low-fat yogurt (27 cals).

\\ This tagine is quite substantial on its own, but for an even bulkier meal, serve with Cauliflower Couscous (page 118; 42 cals) or wholemeal couscous (88 cals per ½ cup cooked).

\\ Top freely with chopped fresh herbs such as parsley, dill and mint (calories negligible).

\\ Keep, covered, in the fridge for up to 3 days. Can also be frozen.

\\ Feed the non-fasters: Multiply ingredients as necessary and serve with buttered couscous.

SWEET & SOUR BEAN & BEETROOT STEW

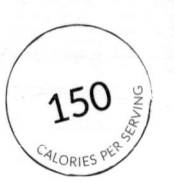

150
CALORIES PER SERVING

Gluten-free \\ Dairy-free \\ Vegan

NUTRITIONAL INFO PER SERVING: 1g fat, of which 0.3g saturates

27g carbohydrate, of which 18g sugars \\ 8g protein \\ 3g salt \\ 11g fibre

---

This is based on a classic borscht that my Ukranian stepmother makes – chunky, rich and immensely satisfying with a thick broth (using tomato juice as well as stock) and the goodness of protein-rich kidney beans and heaps of vegetables. In lieu of the traditional sour cream, add a dollop of low-fat yogurt.

PREP & COOK TIME: **30 MINUTES**

SERVINGS: **2 LARGE**

70g/2½oz/about ½ large carrot
4 spring onions (scallions)
2 celery stalks
½ green pepper
100g/3½oz pickled beetroot, drained
1 garlic clove
250ml/9fl oz/generous 1 cup hot stock
  or water + 1 tsp stock powder

125g/4½oz/¾ cup red kidney beans
  (½ x 400g can, drained)
325ml/11fl oz/1⅓ cups tomato juice
1 tsp agave nectar or honey
sea salt and freshly ground
  black pepper
pinch of cayenne pepper (optional)
50g/1¾oz (about 2 large leaves) Savoy
  cabbage

1. Boil the kettle while you roughly chop the carrot. Put the carrot in a medium saucepan and add the hot stock or water. Bring to the boil, then reduce the heat to a simmer while you roughly chop the remaining veg (including the beetroot) and crush the garlic. After 5 minutes, add the onions, celery, green pepper and garlic to the carrot. Simmer for a further 5 minutes.

2. Add the beetroot, kidney beans, tomato juice and agave or honey to the pan with salt, pepper and cayenne to taste and bring to the boil, then simmer for 5 more minutes while you finely shred the cabbage.

3. Add the cabbage and simmer until tender, about 5 minutes, then serve.

4. Cook for 10 minutes, stirring occasionally, until the veg have softened and the sauce has thickened. Serve.

\\ For the perfect finish, top with a heaped tablespoon of low-fat yogurt (27 cals).

\\ Freely add chopped fresh herbs: dill, parsley or basil (calories negligible).

\\ Keep, covered, in the fridge for up to 3 days. Can also be frozen.

GREEN GUMBO WITH PARMESAN

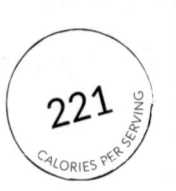

221 CALORIES PER SERVING

Dairy-free \\ Vegan (if Parmesan is omitted)
NUTRITIONAL INFO PER SERVING: 8g fat, of which 3g saturates
26g carbohydrate, of which 7g sugars \\ 11g protein \\ 3g salt \\ 9g fibre

Lashings of Parmesan on a fast day? Yes, you can! This Creole-style green stew, thickened with okra and bulgur wheat or couscous, is crammed to the gills with green veggie goodness and is low-cal enough to welcome Parmesan with open arms (see note about Parmesan, page 33). The Parmesan brings a tangy zeal and a little extra protein, but you could, of course, leave it out and subtract 44 cals per serving. Louisiana hot sauce is optional but darn tasty!

PREP & COOK TIME: **30 MINUTES**
SERVINGS: **2 LARGE**

150g/5½oz okra
100g/3½oz leek
½ green pepper
2 celery sticks
1 garlic clove
2 tsp olive oil
500ml/18fl oz/2 cups boiling water
2 tsp stock powder
50g/1¾oz/5 tbsp bulgur wheat or wholemeal couscous

100g/3½oz cabbage or kale
large handful (about 10g/¼oz) of fresh parsley
leaves stripped from a few fresh thyme stalks, or ½ tsp dried thyme
20g/¾oz Parmesan cheese
1 tbsp white wine vinegar
sea salt and freshly ground black pepper
Louisiana hot sauce (such as Tabasco), to taste

1 Boil the kettle.

2 Slice the tops off the okra, slice thinly and set aside.

3 Chop the leek, green pepper, celery and garlic.

4 Heat a saucepan over a medium heat and add the oil. Add the okra and fry until tinged with gold, about 3 minutes.

5 Add the garlic and fry for a few seconds until fragrant, then pour in the hot water. Add the stock powder and stir.

6 Add the bulgur wheat or couscous, leek, green pepper and celery, return to the boil and simmer for 5 minutes.

7 Meanwhile, shred the cabbage or kale, and chop the parsley, then add to the pan with the thyme. Simmer for 5 more minutes, by which time the bulgur wheat or couscous should be plumped and cooked. Meanwhile, grate the Parmesan.

8 Remove the pan from the heat and stir in the vinegar. Taste the broth and season with salt and pepper.

9 Add hot sauce to each bowl and spoon over the Parmesan.

\\ Keep in an airtight container in the fridge for up to 3 days. Can also be frozen (add hot sauce and Parmesan just before serving).

\\ Feed the non-fasters: A traditional accompaniment for gumbo is cornbread. An easy alternative would be tortilla chips, crusty bread, or garlic bread. Add grated Cheddar and sour cream to each bowl.

HOT & SOUR TOFU BOWL

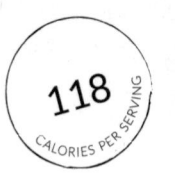

118
CALORIES PER SERVING

Gluten-free (if gluten-free soy sauce is used) \\ Dairy-free \\ Vegan
NUTRITIONAL INFO PER SERVING: 4g fat, of which 0.5g saturates
10g carbohydrate, of which 9g sugars \\ 10g protein \\ 4.2g salt \\ 3g fibre

Health-boosting sauerkraut creates the 'sour' and chilli the 'hot' in this speedy Korean-style soup. Kimchi can be used in place of sauerkraut – check the label to see that it's around 20 calories per 100g and, if you are vegetarian, that it does not contain fish products.

PREP & COOK TIME: **12 MINUTES**
SERVINGS: **1 LARGE**

100g/3½oz fresh firm tofu
125ml/4fl oz/½ cup water
2 tsp seasoned rice vinegar or
   sushi vinegar
1 tbsp dark soy sauce

1 tsp agave nectar or honey
cayenne pepper or chilli flakes, to taste
½ tsp garlic powder or
   1 fresh garlic clove
100g/3½oz/1⅓ cup sauerkraut,
   drained
1 spring onion (scallion)

1. Drain the tofu and wrap in paper towels to absorb excess moisture, then cut into bite-sized cubes.

2. Put the water in a saucepan and add the vinegar, soy sauce, agave or honey, chilli, and garlic (crush in the garlic if using fresh). Bring to the boil, then add the tofu and sauerkraut, and stir.

3. Reduce the heat, cover and simmer gently for 5 minutes. Finely slice the spring onion and scatter over the top. Serve immediately.

\\ Feel free to add 50–100g/1¾–3½oz fresh chopped vegetables such as broccoli, courgette, spinach or chard (20–30 cals) with the tofu, but bear in mind that the acidity of the liquid will make green veggies slightly off-colour.

\\ Best eaten on the same day. Not suitable for freezing.

SWEET & SOUR TOFU & PINEAPPLE

142 CALORIES PER SERVING

Gluten-free (if gluten-free soy sauce is used) \\ Dairy-free \\ Vegan
NUTRITIONAL INFO PER SERVING: 4g fat, of which 0.5g saturates
16g carbohydrate, of which 12g sugars \\ 10g protein \\ 2.7g salt \\ 2g fibre

Tofu just loves to get the chance to soak up all these vibrant Asian flavours with a good balance of sweet, sour, salty and hot. For convenience, use ready-prepared fresh pineapple. Canned pineapple can be used, but make sure it's unsweetened in juice, rather than syrup. This sensational concoction is also fabulous served chilled as a salad.

PREP & COOK TIME: **25 MINUTES**
SERVINGS: **2 MEDIUM**

100g/3½oz/1 medium red onion
2 tbsp dark soy sauce
2 tbsp water
2 tbsp fresh lime juice
1 tsp agave nectar or honey

½ tsp chilli flakes, or to taste
200g/7oz fresh firm tofu, drained and
  wrapped in paper towels
100g/3½oz fresh pineapple
1cm/½in piece fresh ginger
2 garlic cloves
1 tsp cornflour (cornstarch)
1 tsp cold water

1 | Halve and slice the onion. Place in a lidded saucepan with the soy sauce, 2 tbsp water, lime juice, agave or honey, and chilli flakes. Cover and bring to the boil, then simmer for about 5 minutes while you prepare the remaining ingredients.

2 | Cut the tofu into 2cm x 5mm/¾in x ¼in slices. Cut the pineapple into bite-sized chunks. Peel and chop the ginger and crush the garlic.

3 | Add the tofu, pineapple, ginger and garlic to the pan. Return to the boil and simmer for 10 minutes, stirring occasionally – gently, so as not to break up the tofu too much.

4 | Mix the cornflour with 1 tsp cold water and stir into the pan to thicken the liquid, then serve.

\\ Enjoy on its own or with Cauliflower Couscous (page 118; 42 cals) or ½ cup cooked brown rice (108 cals).

\\ Also great with Egg Strand Noodles (page 131) or shirataki noodles (page 116).

\\ Add extra flavour and nutrition by sprinkling with toasted sesame seeds (52 cals per tbsp).

\\ Top freely with chopped fresh coriander and/or chives (calories negligible).

\\ This dish is also delicious served cold as a salad – eat with some crunchy salad leaves or fresh raw bean sprouts.

\\ Keep in an airtight container in the fridge for up to 3 days. Can also be frozen.

\\ Feed the non-fasters: Multiply ingredients as necessary and serve with rice or noodles. Top with toasted cashew nuts.

TERIYAKI TOFU
& ROASTED BROCCOLI

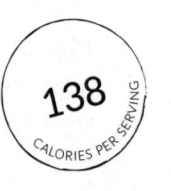

138 CALORIES PER SERVING

Gluten-free (if gluten-free soy sauce is used) \\ Dairy-free \\ Vegan
NUTRITIONAL INFO PER SERVING: 7g fat, of which 0.8g saturates
7g carbohydrate, of which 5g sugars \\ 13g protein \\ 1.4g salt \\ 4g fibre

Mirin – Japanese cooking wine – gives an authentic teriyaki flavour here in tandem with the soy sauce and ginger, but you could use any cooking wine recommended on page 36. Roasting broccoli transforms it into quite a different creature – even using minimum oil. Just whack it all in the oven and enjoy!

PREP & COOK TIME: **30 MINUTES**
SERVINGS: **2 LARGE**

200g/7oz fresh firm tofu
spray oil
1 tbsp dark soy sauce

1 tbsp mirin
1cm/½in piece fresh ginger
200g/7oz broccoli
1 tsp extra-virgin rapeseed oil or
   olive oil

1. Preheat the oven to 220°C/425°F/Gas Mark 7.

2. Pat the tofu dry and cut into 4 slabs about 1cm/½in thick.

3. Line a roasting pan with non-stick baking parchment or non-stick foil. Spray 4 times with spray oil. Lay the tofu on it.

4. In a small bowl, combine the soy sauce and mirin. Peel and finely grate the ginger and stir it through the sauce. Spoon the sauce evenly over the tofu.

5 | Break the broccoli into small florets. (Note: if saving the second portion, use just half the broccoli now.)

6 | Spoon the oil into a zip-seal bag and add the broccoli. Seal the bag and massage the oil all over the broccoli to coat completely.

7 | Arrange the broccoli around the tofu.

8 | Bake for 20–25 minutes, until the edges of the tofu and broccoli are darkened. Serve immediately.

\\ Keep the tofu in an airtight container in the fridge for up to 3 days. It can also be frozen: the texture will change slightly. The broccoli is best enjoyed immediately – steam fresh broccoli to accompany the saved portion.

\\ Feed the non-fasters: Serve with wholegrain rice or noodles.

MIRACULOUSLY RICH HOTPOT

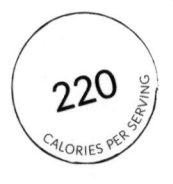

220 CALORIES PER SERVING

Gluten-free \\ Dairy-free \\ Vegan
NUTRITIONAL INFO PER SERVING: 3g fat, of which 0.3g saturates
38g carbohydrate, of which 23g sugars \\ 10g protein \\ 0.8g salt \\ 9g fibre

The miracle? Carrot juice. Used as a stock to cook veggies, it imparts a sweet and satisfying richness, enhanced by spices and dried shiitake mushrooms. If dried are unavailable, use fresh shiitake or other fresh or dried mushrooms, but dried shiitake are a great 5:2 cupboard item, with a host of health benefits and oodles of flavour. They are available from Asian groceries and health food shops. Feel free to vary the other vegetables from the list of suitable ones (page 26). I think this particular combo works amazingly well.

PREP & COOK TIME: **30 MINUTES**
SERVINGS: **2 LARGE**

500ml/18fl oz/generous 2 cups carrot
  juice (fresh or long-life)
4 dried shiitake mushrooms (see intro)
100g/3½oz/1 small–medium turnip
100g/3½oz/1 medium red onion
½ red pepper
100g/3½oz fresh tomatoes

50g/1¾oz green beans
125g/4½oz/¾ cup canned chickpeas
  (½ x 400g can, drained)
2 garlic cloves
handful of fresh basil and/or parsley
½ tsp fennel seeds
about ½ tsp freshly grated nutmeg
cayenne pepper or chilli flakes, to taste
sea salt and freshly ground
  black pepper

1   Put the carrot juice in a saucepan and bring to the boil, then reduce the heat to medium.

2   Meanwhile, break the shiitake mushrooms into small pieces. Rinse and then add to the pan.

3   Prepare the veg and toss them into the pan, in this order: peel and cube the turnip and add. Coarsely chop the red onion, red pepper and tomato and add. Cut the beans into bite-sized pieces and add. Add the chickpeas, crush in the garlic, tear in the herbs, add the fennel seeds, nutmeg, cayenne, if desired, and plenty of salt and pepper.

4   After about 15 minutes, everything should be boiling in the pan.

5   Reduce the heat to a simmer and cook for 10–15 minutes more. Serve.

\\ For a creamy tang, top with a heaped tablespoon of low-fat yogurt (27 cals).

\\ Top freely with chopped fresh herbs such as parsley and basil (calories negligible).

\\ Keep, covered, in the fridge for up to 3 days. Can also be frozen.

\\ Feed the non-fasters: Multiply ingredients as necessary and serve with buttered couscous, rice, crusty bread, or a hot garlic baguette.

SAFFRON CELERIAC AND PUY LENTIL BOWL

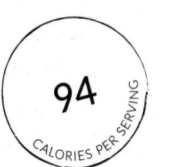

94 CALORIES PER SERVING

Gluten-free \\ Dairy-free \\ Vegan

NUTRITIONAL INFO PER SERVING: 1g fat, of which 0.2g saturates

13g carbohydrate, of which 5g sugars \\ 7g protein \\ 1.5g salt \\ 10g fibre

A few simple ingredients come together to create a subtly flavoured sensation, for less than 100 calories! Celeriac is one of your best friends for fast days – whether cooked or raw, it is low in calories and carbs, intensely flavoured and just as filling as a starchy vegetable. Ready-cooked lentils are a fantastic high-protein convenience food, which can be found in long-life packets and also in cans.

PREP & COOK TIME: **25 MINUTES**

SERVINGS: **2 LARGE**

100g/3½oz leek
200g/7oz celeriac (peeled weight)
250ml/9fl oz/generous 1 cup boiling water

1 tsp stock powder
large pinch of saffron strands
100g/3½oz cooked Puy lentils or other lentils
100g/3½oz ripe cherry tomatoes
sea salt and freshly ground black pepper

1. Boil the kettle while you prepare the leek and celeriac. Slice the leek and cut the celeriac into small cubes. Place them in a lidded saucepan with the water, stock powder and saffron, stir and bring to the boil. Cover and simmer for 10 minutes.

2. Add the lentils and tomatoes to the pan and season with salt and pepper. Simmer for a further 5 minutes and serve.

\\ Enjoy on its own or with a serving of Cauliflower Couscous (page 118; 42 cals), ½ cup cooked brown rice (108 cals), or half a pitta bread (62 cals).

\\ Top freely with chopped fresh coriander or parsley (calories negligible).

\\ For a creamy tang, top with a heaped tablespoon of low-fat yogurt (27 cals).

\\ Keep in an airtight container in the fridge for up to 3 days. Can also be frozen.

\\ Feed the non-fasters: Accompany with rice, couscous, or crusty bread, and top with crème fraîche.

SWEET POTATO & PALM HEART CASSEROLE

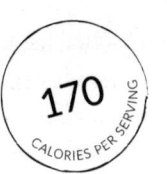

170 CALORIES PER SERVING

Gluten-free \\ Dairy-free \\ Vegan (if Parmesan omitted)

NUTRITIONAL INFO PER SERVING: 4g fat, of which 2g saturates

26g carbohydrate, of which 7g sugars \\ 8g protein \\ 1.5g salt \\ 7g fibre

---

Here's a lovely winter warmer using fast-day friendly palm hearts to fantastic effect, in tandem with sweet potato and Parmesan (see note about Parmesan, page 33).

PREP & COOK TIME: **30 MINUTES**
SERVINGS: **2 MEDIUM**

100g/3½oz leek
200g/7oz sweet potato
  (unpeeled weight)
250ml/9fl oz/generous 1 cup boiling
  water

1 tsp stock powder
200g/7oz palm hearts
  (approx. 1 can, drained)
sea salt and freshly ground
  black pepper
20g/¾oz Parmesan cheese

1 Boil the kettle while you slice the leek and peel the sweet potato and cut into chunks.

2 Place both in a lidded saucepan with the boiling water and stock powder. Stir, cover, bring to the boil, and simmer gently for about 10–15 minutes, checking from time to time, until the potato is soft.

3 Meanwhile, slice the palm hearts and grate the Parmesan. Heat the grill to high.

4 | Much or all of the water may have been absorbed – if so, add a few more splashes to the pan to stop it sticking; otherwise, strain the mixture, (saving the stock for a virtually calorie-free savoury hot drink later on) and return the leeks and sweet potatoes to the pan. Add the palm hearts to the pan. Stir until heated through, crushing the sweet potato lightly, then remove from the heat and season with salt and pepper.

5 | Scoop the contents of the pan into 1 medium or 2 individual casserole dishes (if saving the second portion, just leave it to cool, then chill or freeze; finish under the grill just before eating).

6 | Sprinkle with Parmesan and place under the grill for 3–4 minutes, until golden and bubbly.

\\ Accompany with a mixed-leaf salad and sliced ripe tomatoes dressed with sea salt, pepper and fresh lemon juice or balsamic vinegar (about 50 cals).

\\ Top freely with chopped fresh parsley (calories negligible). Or add a spicy kick with some cayenne pepper or chilli sauce.

\\ Keep in an airtight container in the fridge for up to 3 days. Keep the Parmesan in a separate container; sprinkle over and grill just before serving. Can also be frozen.

\\ Feed the non-fasters: Accompany with a mixed-leaf and tomato salad topped with walnuts or toasted pine nuts and a balsamic vinaigrette made with good olive oil. Top each casserole portion with crème fraîche.

SOUTH INDIAN MANGO CURRY

137 CALORIES PER SERVING

Gluten-free

NUTRITIONAL INFO PER SERVING: 3g fat, of which 0.8g saturates
24g carbohydrate, of which 20g sugars \\ 4g protein \\ 0.1g salt \\ 4g fibre

South Indian curries are usually quick, often fruity, and always exploding with flavour. This sweet and saucy curry tastes as gorgeous as it looks. Use ready-prepared fresh mango chunks for speed and ease. If cutting your own, even a slightly under-ripe mango works here – just peel, slice off the 'cheeks' either side of the stone, and cut into chunks – 2 cheeks will be roughly 200g. If you have access to some fresh or frozen curry leaves, by all means throw them in as well.

PREP & COOK TIME: **25 MINUTES**
SERVINGS: **2 MEDIUM**

1 small fresh chilli or a large pinch of dried chilli flakes
1cm/½in piece fresh ginger
2 garlic cloves
3 spring onions (scallions)
100g/3½oz tomatoes
200g/7oz prepared fresh mango chunks

1 tsp sunflower oil
1 tsp black or brown mustard seeds
½ tsp turmeric
½ tsp cumin seeds
75ml/2½fl oz/5 tbsp water
sea salt and freshly ground black pepper
125g/4½oz/½ cup low-fat yogurt
2 tsp cornflour (cornstarch)

1 Slit the chilli in half or slice roughly. Peel the ginger and chop or grate it. Peel the garlic. Slice the spring onions, cut the tomatoes into chunky pieces, and cut the mango into bite-sized chunks if necessary.

2 Heat a large non-stick frying pan over a medium–high heat and add the oil and mustard seeds. As soon the mustard seeds start to pop, which should happen almost immediately if the pan is hot, remove the pan from the heat and add the turmeric, cumin, chilli and ginger. Crush the garlic into the pan, return the pan to a medium heat, and stir for a few seconds until fragrant.

3 Add the onions, tomatoes, mango and water with a generous seasoning of salt and pepper, and cook for about 3 minutes, until the tomato softens.

4 Measure the yogurt into a small bowl and beat in the cornflour. Add to the pan, stirring thoroughly until the sauce turns yellow and just starts to bubble, then remove from the heat. Eat immediately.

\\ Enjoy on its own or with Cauliflower Couscous (page 118; 42 cals), or ½ cup cooked brown rice (108 cals), or half a pitta bread (62 cals). For extra protein, top with a quartered hard-boiled egg (72 cals).

\\ Top with chopped fresh coriander for an authentic finish (calories negligible).

\\ Keep in an airtight container in the fridge for up to 3 days. Can also be frozen. Reheat in the microwave; stir very thoroughly, as the sauce might curdle slightly on reheating, but it is still delicious.

\\ Feed the non-fasters: Accompany with cooked brown or basmati rice and/or naan bread.

SOUTH INDIAN EGG & COCONUT CURRY

198 CALORIES PER SERVING

Gluten-free

NUTRITIONAL INFO PER SERVING: 12g fat, of which 5g saturates

13g carbohydrate, of which 8g sugars \\ 11g protein \\ 0.3g salt \\ 3g fibre

---

A delectable variation of my Mango Curry (page 106), using boiled eggs and dried coconut.

PREP & COOK TIME: **25 MINUTES**

SERVINGS: **2 MEDIUM**

2 eggs
1 small fresh chilli or a large pinch of dried chilli flakes
1cm/½in piece fresh ginger
2 garlic cloves
3 spring onions (scallions)
200g/7oz tomatoes
1 tsp sunflower oil

1 tsp black or brown mustard seeds
½ tsp turmeric
½ tsp cumin seeds
2 tbsp (about 12g) unsweetened desiccated coconut
3 tbsp water
sea salt and freshly ground black pepper
125g/4½oz/½ cup low-fat yogurt
2 tsp cornflour (cornstarch)

1 Put the eggs in a small pan and cover with cold water. Bring to the boil and cook for 7 minutes, then drain and rinse under cold water until cool.

2 Meanwhile, prepare the other ingredients. Slit the chilli in half or slice roughly. Peel the ginger and chop or grate it. Peel the garlic. Slice the spring onions, and cut the tomatoes into chunky pieces.

3   Heat a large non-stick frying pan over a medium–high heat and add the oil and mustard seeds. As soon the mustard seeds start to pop, which should happen almost immediately if the pan is hot, remove the pan from the heat and add the turmeric, cumin, coconut, chilli and ginger. Crush the garlic into the pan, return the pan to a medium heat, and stir for a few seconds until fragrant.

4   Add the onions and water with a generous seasoning of salt and pepper, and cook for about 2 minutes, until the onion softens. Meanwhile, peel the eggs if cooked and cooled.

5   Add the tomatoes and whole eggs to the pan and stir until the tomatoes start to soften, about 3 minutes.

6   Measure the yogurt into a small bowl and beat in the cornflour. Add to the pan, stirring thoroughly until the sauce turns yellow and just starts to bubble, then remove from the heat. Serve one egg in its sauce per serving. Eat immediately.

\\ Enjoy on its own or with Cauliflower Couscous (page 118; 42 cals), ½ cup cooked brown rice (108 cals), or half a pitta bread (62 cals).

\\ Top with chopped fresh coriander for an authentic finish (calories negligible).

\\ Keep in an airtight container in the fridge for up to 3 days. Can also be frozen. Reheat in the microwave; stir very thoroughly, as the sauce might curdle slightly on reheating, but it is still delicious.

\\ Feed the non-fasters: Accompany with cooked brown or basmati rice and/or naan bread.

SOUTH INDIAN TOFU & MUSHROOM CURRY

147 CALORIES PER SERVING

Gluten-free \\ Dairy-free \\ Vegan

NUTRITIONAL INFO PER SERVING: **8g** fat, of which **1g** saturates

4g carbohydrate, of which **3g** sugars \\ **14g** protein \\ **1.2g** salt \\ **2g** fibre

---

Tofu is not a traditional South Indian ingredient – paneer or curd cheese would be more appropriate here, but, alas, not an ingredient for fast days! Low-fat and high-protein tofu works a treat instead and absorbs all the exotic spicy sauce.

PREP & COOK TIME: **25 MINUTES**

SERVINGS: **2 MEDIUM**

300g/10½oz fresh firm tofu
1 small fresh chilli or a large pinch of
  dried chilli flakes
1cm/½in piece fresh ginger
2 garlic cloves
3 spring onions (scallions)
100g/3½oz tomatoes

100g/3½oz chestnut (cremini) or
  white mushrooms
1 tsp sunflower oil
1 tsp black or brown mustard seeds
½ tsp turmeric
½ tsp cumin seeds
3 tbsp water + 1 tsp stock powder
sea salt and freshly ground
  black pepper
1 tsp fresh lemon juice

1. Drain the tofu and wrap in paper towels. Set aside.

2. Slit the chilli in half or slice roughly. Peel the ginger and chop or grate it. Peel the garlic. Slice the spring onions, cut the tomatoes into chunky pieces, and slice the mushrooms thickly.

3 │ Heat a large non-stick frying pan over a medium–high heat and add the oil and mustard seeds. As soon the mustard seeds start to pop, which should happen almost immediately if the pan is hot, remove the pan from the heat and add the turmeric, cumin, chilli and ginger. Crush garlic into the pan, return the pan to the heat, and stir for a few seconds until fragrant.

4 │ Add the water and stock powder, and stir until bubbling.

5 │ Add the onions, tomato and mushrooms with a generous seasoning of salt and pepper, and stir.

6 │ Cut the tofu into cubes and add to the pan, or simply break in the tofu in fairly large chunks. Cook for about 10 minutes, stirring frequently, until the liquid is absorbed and the tofu and mushrooms are tinged with gold.

7 │ Remove the pan from the heat and stir in the lemon juice, then serve.

\\ Enjoy on its own or with Cauliflower Couscous (page 118; 42 cals), or ½ cup cooked brown rice (108 cals), or half a pitta bread (62 cals).

\\ Serve with a tangy dollop of low-fat yogurt (27 cals for a heaped tbsp).

\\ Top with chopped fresh coriander for an authentic finish (calories negligible).

\\ Keep in an airtight container in the fridge for up to 2 days. Can also be frozen. Reheat in the microwave.

\\ Feed the non-fasters: Accompany with cooked brown or basmati rice and/or naan bread.

CHAPTER 5
FLAVOUR BOMBS

THE RECIPES in the second part of this chapter create intense flavours using low-calorie ingredients; they can be added to various simple meals for a satisfying composition with minimum effort. Your basic, bulky, fast-day meals – what I call 'plain flavour canvases' – can be transformed by the introduction of a flavour bomb – KAPOW!

The first part of the chapter suggests some 'plain flavour canvases', such as Cauliflower Couscous and variations (page 118), and some low-cal ways to go to work on an egg (page 126–133). You might also like to try:

- A bowl of steamed mixed veg and tofu, with or without a small portion of rice, bulgur wheat, quinoa, or low-fat ramen noodles, dressed with a little soy sauce and lemon juice.

- A plate of mixed salad dressed with rice vinegar or lemon juice, with light cottage cheese, a hard-boiled egg or fresh firm tofu.

- A baked potato or sweet potato, or Crushed Potatoes (page 125), with low-fat yogurt or cottage cheese, plus cooked or raw veg or salad.

- Shirataki noodles (see pages 34 and 116).

Now add a flavour bomb from this chapter of sauces and tasty morsels – and relish your meal without piling on the calories.

PLAIN FLAVOUR
CANVASES

SHIRATAKI NOODLES

These rather peculiar jelly-textured noodles (also sold in 'rice' and 'pasta' shapes) definitely need some TLC to make them palatable. They are completely flavourless, but absorb flavours well. As for texture, they are quite firm and won't soften even if you boil them for hours (I've tried). Boiling them in salted water or stock, however, lets the flavour in.

One thing that doesn't do them any favours is drying them out. Some people recommend draining and rinsing them and then dry-frying them in a non-stick pan. I find this makes them tougher – like eating a bowlful of rubber bands. And they get stuck in your teeth. Not so nice!

Whichever preparation method you prefer or shape you choose, it's universally agreed that they need to be rinsed – a lot. They may appear ready-to-eat in their watery packet, but once you release them, you'll understand why. They smell odd – downright fishy. Don't worry – this is soon remedied. Just follow these instructions for preparation and cooking. One packet is usually enough for one generous or two small servings.

1. Boil a small amount of water in the kettle for cooking the noodles.

2. Place a fine sieve in the sink. Use scissors to open the packet of noodles over the sieve and drain away the liquid.

3. Rinse the noodles under the tap running with hand-hot water, tossing them well, for 1–2 minutes, until there is no perceptible odour.

4. Place them in a small saucepan and just cover with boiling water. Bring to the boil, adding a generous dose of salt, or a teaspoonful of stock powder or a stock cube. Simmer for 5 minutes or more (it's impossible to overcook them – longer cooking will allow them to develop more flavour).

5 Drain and serve.

6 If saving for later, the noodles can now be cooled and stored in an airtight container in the fridge for up to 3 days. They can also be eaten cold.

Serving options:

- To serve with a warm sauce, stir the cooked noodles through the sauce in the pan and either simmer them together for a few minutes or allow them to stand together for several minutes to absorb flavour further.

- To serve as a bed for a recipe, or as an accompaniment to steamed veg or tofu, dress the noodles by stirring through a little soy or teriyaki sauce (if they are not sufficiently salty already), or Thai chilli sauce such as Sriracha, or add a squeeze of fresh lemon or lime juice.

- For a Mediterranean theme, add some fresh thyme sprigs and a few crumbled porcini mushrooms when boiling the noodles.

CAULIFLOWER COUSCOUS

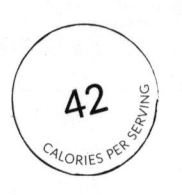

Gluten-free \\ Dairy-free \\ Vegan

NUTRITIONAL INFO PER SERVING: 1g fat, of which 0.2g saturates

4g carbohydrate, of which 3g sugars \\ 5g protein \\ trace salt \\ 3g fibre

This might be the most versatile basic element in your 5:2 regime, period. It is scarcely recognizable as a vegetable in flavour, and certainly neither in appearance nor texture. Like the wheat-based couscous it mimics, it has fabulous absorption properties, so it's great with anything saucy. On fast days, you can just ignore calorific, slow-cooking grains and gorge on this instead.

It is simply raw cauliflower whizzed to couscous-like proportions, then steamed in the microwave. It can be used as a bed for just about anything and is the perfect way to bulk out a meal, contributing minimal calories and bringing all the wonderful health benefits of this regal vegetable, including cancer-fighting phytonutrients.

PREP & COOK TIME: **10 MINUTES**

SERVINGS: **2 LARGE**

250g/9oz cauliflower

sea salt

1 Break the cauliflower into florets, wash and drain.

2 Place in a food processor and whizz until reduced to crumbs the size of couscous.

3 Scrape into a microwave-safe container and sprinkle with salt, distributing it evenly with your fingertips. (No need to add water.)

4   Cover and cook for 3 minutes, then stand for 2 minutes. (Microwaves vary: the cauliflower should be cooked through.) Serve.

\\ Keep in an airtight container in the fridge for up to 3 days. Can also be frozen. From frozen, place in a microwave-safe container and heat on high power for 1 minute. Break up with a fork and cook for another 2 minutes, fluff and serve.

CHARGRILLED CAULIFLOWER SLAB

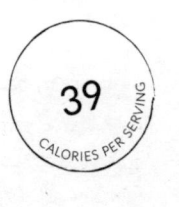

39
CALORIES PER SERVING

Gluten-free \\ Dairy-free \\ Vegan
NUTRITIONAL INFO PER SERVING: 1g fat, of which 0.3g saturates
3g carbohydrate, of which 3g sugars \\ 4g protein \\ trace salt \\ 2g fibre

Here's another simple treatment for cauliflower to be used as a plain flavour canvas. Chargrilling imparts a lovely smoky flavour. You'll only get one 'slab' per cauliflower – a cross-section of its fattest part, which weighs about 100g – so use the rest for Cauliflower Couscous or save the florets for steaming.

PREP & COOK TIME: **12 MINUTES**
SERVINGS: **1 LARGE**

1 medium cauliflower
spray oil
sea salt and freshly ground
black pepper

1   Heat a ridged grill pan over a high heat until extremely hot.

2   Cut a 1cm/½in thick slab through the middle of the cauliflower, cutting down through the stem. Save the remainder for another use.

3 │ Spray the cauli slab about 3 times with spray oil and place oil-side down in the grill pan. Spray the top with 3 more sprays of oil and season with salt and pepper.

4 │ After about 4–5 minutes, the bottom should be striped with black. Use tongs to flip over the cauli slab. Season the top with salt and pepper and cook until striped to your liking, about 4–5 minutes. Serve as a base for your chosen topping.

\\ Serve with any of the South Indian curries (pages 106–111), with Creamy Paprika Mushrooms (page 80), Smoky Spanish Stir-fry (page 72), the lentil mixture from Sweet Lentil Cabbage Wraps (page 82), Almond & Tomato Sauce (page 155), or Creamy Spiked Spinach (page 136).

CAULIFLOWER PARMESAN PANCAKES

184 CALORIES PER SERVING

Gluten-free

NUTRITIONAL INFO PER SERVING: 13g fat, of which 4g saturates
2g carbohydrate, of which 2g sugars \\ 14g protein \\ 0.4g salt \\ 2g fibre

Apart from being a great grain substitute, Cauliflower Couscous (page 118) makes a fabulous ingredient. See also Raw Cauliflower & Feta Tabbouleh (page 44).

PREP & COOK TIME: 15 MINUTES, PLUS 10 FOR MAKING CAULIFLOWER COUSCOUS
SERVINGS: **2 LARGE**

200g/7oz/about 1½ cups loosely packed Cauliflower Couscous, cooled

20g/¾oz/about 4 tbsp freshly grated Parmesan cheese
2 eggs
freshly ground black pepper
2 tsp sunflower oil

1   In a bowl, beat together the cauliflower, Parmesan and eggs, and season well with pepper.

2   Heat a non-stick frying pan over a medium heat and add 1 tsp oil. Spoon in half of the batter to make 4 pancakes. Smooth the tops.

3   Cook until deep golden on the bottom, then carefully flip over and cook the other side – this can be a bit tricky and you may need to use two spatulas. Cook until golden. Remove to a plate.

4   Add the remaining 1 tsp oil to the pan. Cook 4 more pancakes, then serve or reserve.

\\ Serve with Napoli Sauce (page 151) or Puttanesca Sauce (page 153). Finish with extra freshly grated Parmesan (22 cals per tbsp). Serve with a crunchy salad.

\\ Make mini pizzas: top with a spoonful of low-calorie pizza sauce or Napoli Sauce (page 153) and finish with reduced-fat grated mozzarella or grated Parmesan, then cook in a preheated oven at 200°C/400°F/Gas Mark 6 until the cheese is golden and bubbly.

\\ The pancakes can be kept in a resealable bag in the fridge for up to 3 days. Reheat in a preheated oven at 200°C/400°F/Gas Mark 6 for about 5–7 minutes. They can also be frozen – reheat from frozen in the oven as above for about 10 minutes.

PERFECT POTATOES & SWEET POTATOES

Good old potatoes, and their botanically unrelated cousins sweet potatoes, are often shunned by the anti-carb diet brigade, but they do provide a perfect canvas for a variety of flavours and textures. They are filling, low-fat vegetables, which just about everybody loves, and can fit snugly in the 5:2 diet in moderation, especially if eaten with the skin on for maximum nutrition. Some studies have cited baked potatoes as an appetite suppressant.

PERFECT JACKETS

You'll need about an hour of forward planning for oven-baked jacket potatoes or sweet potatoes with a lovely crisp skin. Or they can be ready to eat in under 10 minutes in the microwave. Larger ones can be cut down to the desired weight.

OVEN-BAKED JACKETS

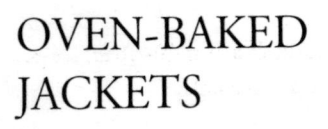

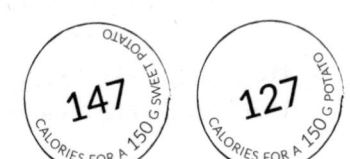

Gluten-free \\ Dairy-free \\ Vegan

NUTRITIONAL INFO PER SERVING: (150g potato) 2g fat, of which 0.1g saturates
24g carbohydrate, of which 0.9g sugars \\ 3g protein \\ 0g salt \\ 3g fibre
(150g sweet potato) 2g fat, of which 0.3g saturates
30g carbohydrate, of which 8g sugars \\ 2g protein \\ 0.2g salt \\ 5g fibre

PREP & COOK TIME: **45–55 MINUTES**
SERVINGS: **1 MEDIUM**

1 potato or sweet potato, weighing
    150–200g/5½–7oz
a few drops of oil
    (any cooking oil is fine)
sea salt, ideally flakes

1 | Preheat the oven to 200°C/400°F/Gas Mark 6. (Note: Sweet potatoes may seep their sugary syrup while baking, so you may wish to place a piece of foil or a baking sheet on the bottom rack of the oven.)

2 | If the potato is dirty, scrub and dry well. Otherwise, merely wipe with a damp cloth, as adding extra moisture impedes the crisping of the skin.

3 | Working over a chopping board, stab the potato several times with a fork.

4 | Place a few drops of oil in the palm of your hand and rub it all over the potato.

5 | Grab a large pinch of sea salt and rub it all over the potato. Press and roll the potato in any salt that has fallen onto the board.

6 | Place it in the oven, directly on the top rack. Bake for 40–50 minutes. Using tongs, turn halfway through cooking if possible.

7 | Remove from the oven with tongs and drive a sharp knife into the centre to ensure it is soft throughout; if not, cook for a few more minutes until done, then serve immediately.

MICROWAVE-BAKED JACKETS

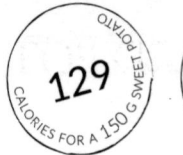

Gluten-free \\ Dairy-free \\ Vegan

NUTRITIONAL INFO PER SERVING: (150g potato) 0.3g fat, of which 0g saturates
24g carbohydrate, of which 0.9g sugars \\ 3g protein \\ 0g salt \\ 3g fibre
(150g sweet potato) 0.5g fat, of which 0.1g saturates
30g carbohydrate, of which 8g sugars \\ 2g protein \\ 0.2g salt \\ 5g fibre

---

PREP & COOK TIME: **7–8 MINUTES**

SERVINGS: **1 MEDIUM**

1 potato or sweet potato, weighing
150–200g/5½–7oz

1. Scrub the potato and pat dry.

2. Stab the potato several times with a fork.

3. Wrap in a paper towel and place it in the microwave, on a microwave-safe plate. Cook on high power for 3 minutes.

4. Using tongs, turn the potato over and cook for a further 2 minutes for 150g, 3 minutes for 200g.

5. Stand for 1 minute.

6. Remove the potato with tongs and drive a sharp knife into the centre to ensure it is soft throughout; if not, cook until done, a minute at a time, then serve immediately.

CRUSHED POTATOES

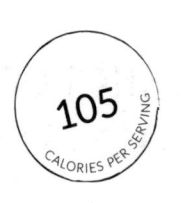

105
CALORIES PER SERVING

Gluten-free \\ Dairy-free \\ Vegan
NUTRITIONAL INFO PER SERVING: 0.5g fat. of which 0.1g saturates
22g carbohydrate, of which 2g sugars \\ 3g protein \\ 0g salt \\ 2g fibre

---

This is an utterly gorgeous and ludicrously simple treatment of ordinary potatoes, especially small new potatoes, though any potato will do. You can boil and crush sweet potatoes too, but leave out the vinegar.

PREP & COOK TIME: **20 MINUTES**
SERVINGS: **2 MEDIUM**

300g/10½oz new or salad potatoes, or
    regular potatoes
salt
1 tbsp best white wine vinegar

1 Scrub the potatoes and cut into chunks.

2 Place in a saucepan and add enough cold water to cover.

3 Place over a high heat and add quite a lot of salt – it should be as briny as seawater.

4 Cover the pan and bring to the boil, then reduce the heat and simmer for 10–15 minutes, until tender throughout.

5 Drain thoroughly – leave to drain for a couple of minutes.

6 Return the potatoes to the pan and add the vinegar. Using a fork, stir and crush the potatoes to incorporate the vinegar, but don't mash completely. Serve hot.

ONE-EGG OMELETTE

74

CALORIES PER SERVING

Gluten-free \\ Dairy-free

NUTRITIONAL INFO PER SERVING: 6g fat, of which 1g saturates

0g carbohydrate, of which 0g sugars \\ 6g protein \\ 0.2g salt \\ 0g fibre

---

Here's how to make a crêpe-thin omelette to be stuffed with the warm filling of your choice (see suggestions below). A high-quality non-stick pan is an imperative bit of kit for 5:2 (see page 20). A 25cm/10in pan is the ideal size for cooking for one or two, and works perfectly for this slim, elegant omelette. Because of the quick cooking time, the chosen filling should be cooked or warmed through before stuffing the omelette.

PREP & COOK TIME: **7 MINUTES**

SERVINGS: **1 MEDIUM**

1 egg

1 tbsp water

sea salt and freshly ground
   black pepper

spray oil

1. In a small bowl, beat together the egg, water and seasoning. Beat until well mixed but not frothy.

2. Heat a non-stick frying pan over a low heat. Spray 4 times with spray oil.

3. Pour in the egg mixture and swirl to coat, then place on the heat. After about a minute, swirl again to spread out the mixture and to cook evenly, forming a crêpe-thin omelette.

4 | Cook for 4–5 minutes, until the top is set. The bottom should be set but not too brown. (If the bottom is browning faster than the top is setting, you may wish to pop the pan under a hot grill to finish setting the egg.)

5 | Gently dislodge the omelette from the pan by carefully loosening the sides with a spatula, and slide it out of the pan onto a plate.

6 | Place your warm filling on half of the omelette and fold over. Serve.

Filling suggestions:

* Creamy Spiked Spinach (page 136)

* Caramelized Artichokes (page 138)

* Instant Garlic Mushrooms (page 135)

* Puttanesca Sauce (page 153)

* Steamed or sautéed veg such as broccoli, courgettes, peppers and mushrooms

SESAME OMELETTE ROLL

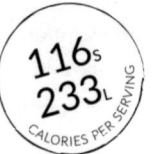

116s
233L
CALORIES PER SERVING

Gluten-free (if gluten-free soy sauce is used) \\ Dairy-free
NUTRITIONAL INFO PER SERVING: (1 large serving) 18g fat, of which 4g saturates
1g carbohydrate, of which 1g sugars \\ 15g protein \\ 1.3g salt \\ 1g fibre

---

PREP & COOK TIME: **15 MINUTES**
SERVINGS: **1 LARGE OR 2 SMALL**

1 tbsp sesame seeds
2 eggs

1 tsp light soy sauce
2 tsp sweet cooking wine (page 36),
 or water
spray oil

---

1 | Heat a non-stick frying pan over a medium heat. Add the sesame seeds to the dry pan and cook, stirring frequently, until golden and popping. Remove from the heat and turn the heat to low. Tip the sesame seeds onto a plate to cool.

2 | Return the pan to the low heat. Preheat the grill to high.

3 | In a small bowl, beat together the eggs, sesame seeds, soy sauce, and wine or water. Beat until well mixed but not frothy.

4 | Heat a non-stick frying pan over a low heat. Spray 4 times with spray oil.

5 | Pour in the egg mixture and swirl to coat, then place on the heat. After about a minute, swirl again to spread out the mixture and to cook evenly.

6 | Cook for 4–5 minutes, until the bottom is set but not too brown.

7 | Pop the pan under the grill until the top is just set, 30 seconds to a minute.

8 | Gently dislodge the omelette from the pan by carefully loosening the sides with a spatula, and slide it out of the pan onto a plate.

9 | When cool enough to handle, roll up, cut into segments and serve. (Can also be served cold.)

\\ Keep in the fridge, well covered, for up to 3 days. Reheat briefly in the microwave. Not suitable for freezing.

INDIAN OMELETTE ROLL

100s
189L
CALORIES PER SERVING

Gluten-free \\ Dairy-free
NUTRITIONAL INFO PER SERVING: (1 large serving) 13g fat, of which 3g saturates
3g carbohydrate, of which 2g sugars \\ 13g protein \\ 0.4g salt \\ 0.6g fibre

PREP & COOK TIME: **15 MINUTES**
SERVINGS: **1 LARGE OR 2 SMALL**

25g/1oz/½ small red onion
1 small red chilli
1cm/½in piece fresh ginger
small handful of fresh coriander
  (cilantro)

1 small garlic clove, or ¼ tsp garlic
  powder or granules
2 eggs
sea salt and freshly ground
  black pepper
½ tsp sunflower or extra-virgin
  rapeseed oil
1 tsp black or brown mustard seeds

1 | Finely chop the onion and chilli and set aside.

2 | Peel and grate the ginger and place in a small bowl. Chop the coriander and add to the ginger. Crush in the garlic or add the garlic powder. Add the eggs with some salt and pepper, and beat the mixture well.

3 | Heat a non-stick frying pan over a medium–high heat. Add the oil and mustard seeds and, as soon as they start to pop, add the onion and chilli. Cook, stirring frequently, until the onion is golden, about 2 minutes, then remove the pan from the heat.

4 | Scrape the contents of the pan into the egg mixture. Return the pan to a low heat. Preheat the grill to high.

5 | Pour the egg mixture into the pan and swirl to coat, then place on the heat. After about a minute, swirl again to spread out the mixture so it cooks evenly.

6 | Cook for 3–4 minutes, until the bottom is set but not too brown.

7 | Pop the pan under the grill until the top is just set, 30 seconds to a minute.

8 | Gently dislodge the omelette from the pan by carefully loosening the sides with a spatula, and slide it out of the pan onto a plate.

9 | When cool enough to handle, roll up, cut into segments and serve.

\\ Keep in the fridge, well covered, for up to 3 days. Reheat briefly in the microwave. Not suitable for freezing.

EGG STRAND NOODLES

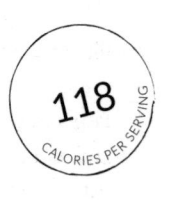

118

CALORIES PER SERVING

Gluten-free \\ Dairy-free

NUTRITIONAL INFO PER SERVING: 8g fat. of which 2g saturates

0.4g carbohydrate, of which 0.4g sugars \\ 9g protein \\ 0.3g salt \\ 0g fibre

---

Your very own homemade all-egg noodles, done in under 30 minutes! Essentially these are super-thin omelettes sliced into noodles. They aren't massively lower in calories than regular noodles, but they consist mostly of protein and are virtually carb-free, meaning you'll stay fuller for longer.

PREP & COOK TIME: **22 MINUTES**

SERVINGS: **2 MEDIUM**

3 eggs

large pinch of sea salt

1 tbsp sweet cooking wine (page 36)

2 tbsp water

spray oil

1 | Place a non-stick frying pan over a low–medium heat.

2 | Combine the eggs with the salt, wine and water, and beat until well mixed but not frothy.

3 | Spray the pan 2 or 3 times with spray oil. (Alternatively, brush with ½ tsp vegetable oil.)

4 | Pour one quarter of the egg mixture into the pan and swirl to coat, making a very thin, even layer.

5 | Leave the egg to cook until completely dry on top, about 4–5 minutes.

6　Loosen the egg with a spatula and gently transfer to a plate to cool (no need to flip over). Don't worry too much if it rips or buckles, but do spread out flat on the plate.

7　Repeat with the remaining egg mixture, stacking the egg sheets as you go.

8　Once cool enough to handle, roll up the four stacked egg sheets. Slice thinly crosswise into ½cm/¼in-wide strips.

9　Loosen and serve hot or cold as noodles.

\\　Keep in an airtight container in the fridge for up to 3 days. Can also be frozen; reheat in the microwave.

PERFECT POACHED EGGS

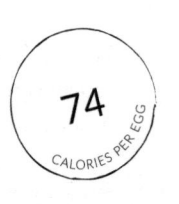

74

CALORIES PER EGG

Gluten-free \\ Dairy-free

NUTRITIONAL INFO PER SERVING: 6g fat, of which 1g saturates

0g carbohydrate, of which 0g sugars \\ 6g protein \\ 0.2g salt \\ 0g fibre

---

Here's my foolproof method for poaching eggs, using a lidded non-stick frying pan, a teacup, and a few minutes longer than your traditional poaching method.

PREP & COOK TIME: **10 MINUTES**

1–4 eggs, as required
½ tsp white wine vinegar
sea salt and freshly ground
black pepper

1 | Bring a 2cm/¾in depth of water to the boil in a large, lidded non-stick frying pan. Reduce the heat to a low simmer. Add the vinegar.

2 | One at a time, carefully break each egg into a cup, then slide the egg into the water. Simmer, covered, for 2 minutes.

3 | Turn off the heat and keep the eggs in the water for 5 minutes. They will then be perfectly cooked if you like the yolk slightly runny. If you prefer a well-done yolk, put the pan back on the heat for 1–2 minutes, until cooked to your liking.

4 | Place a couple of layers of paper towels on a plate. Lift the eggs from the pan with a slotted spoon or spatula and dry briefly on the paper, then serve immediately, seasoning with salt and pepper as desired.

THE FLAVOUR BOMBS

INSTANT GARLIC MUSHROOMS

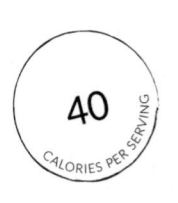

40
CALORIES PER SERVING

Gluten-free \\ Dairy-free \\ Vegan
NUTRITIONAL INFO PER SERVING: 4g fat, of which 0.3g saturates
0.4g carbohydrate, of which 0.2g sugars \\ 2g protein \\ 0.6g salt \\ 2g fibre

OK, almost instant – all done in just a few minutes. You'll need a resealable sandwich bag for coating the mushrooms – the oil is rubbed inside the bag first so every last drop then gets absorbed by the mushrooms, followed by the seasoning. The faithful microwave cooks the mushrooms to juicy perfection – but if you are not a microwave fan, you can bake these in foil in a 220°C/425°F/Gas Mark 7 oven for 20–30 minutes. I've tried both methods and I think the 2-minute microwave method is best for ease and speed, giving juicy mushrooms with a delicious gravy.

PREP & COOK TIME: **7 MINUTES**
SERVINGS: **1 LARGE**

1 tsp extra-virgin rapeseed oil,
    sunflower oil or toasted sesame oil

100g/3½oz chestnut (cremini)
    mushrooms
⅛ tsp fine salt
½ tsp garlic powder or granules
black pepper

1. Open the resealable bag and spoon in the oil. Seal and rub the oil inside the bag.

2. Add the mushrooms, seal, and shake and rub gently to coat the mushrooms all over: they should absorb just about every last drop of oil.

3. Add the salt, garlic powder and pepper, seal and shake gently to coat.

4. Empty the mushrooms into a microwaveable container, cover, leaving an air vent, and microwave on high power for 1 minute. Shake gently, then microwave for 1 minute more.

5. Stand for a minute or so and eat with all the juices.

\\ Use this flavour bomb:
- As a filling for a One-Egg Omelette (page 126).
- Alongside a small jacket potato dressed with low-fat yogurt or cottage cheese.
- With a bowl of steamed vegetables, tofu and low-fat or shirataki noodles (page 116) seasoned with soy sauce and fresh lemon juice.

CREAMY SPIKED SPINACH

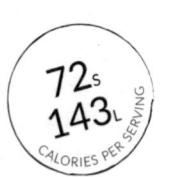

72 s
143 L
CALORIES PER SERVING

Gluten-free

NUTRITIONAL INFO PER SERVING: (1 large serving) 5g fat, of which 1g saturates 17g carbohydrate, of which 9g sugars \\ 8g protein \\ 0.5g salt \\ 3g fibre

Wilted young spinach in a lemony, garlicky, chilli-spiked yogurt-based sauce adds high-impact flavour and superfood goodness to just about anything. One of my favourite fast-day treats.

PREP & COOK TIME: **20 MINUTES**
SERVINGS: **2 SMALL OR 1 LARGE**

100g/3½oz young spinach, washed
100g/3½oz/scant ½ cup low-fat yogurt
1 unwaxed lemon
2 tsp cornflour (cornstarch)

sea salt and freshly ground
  black pepper
1 garlic clove
1 small red chilli or ½ tsp chilli flakes,
  or to taste
1 tsp olive oil

1. Roughly chop the spinach – this can be done quickly and easily by snipping with scissors in the bag or bowl.

2. Measure the yogurt into a small bowl. Wash the lemon well and grate the zest over the bowl of yogurt, taking care not to remove any of the pith. Squeeze the juice and add 2 tsp to the bowl, then beat in the cornflour. Season generously with salt and pepper, and set aside.

3. Peel and chop the garlic and chop or snip the chilli.

4. Heat a lidded saucepan over a low heat and add the oil. Add the garlic and chilli, and fry for about 1 minute, until fragrant, then add the spinach and stir well.

5. Cover the pan and allow the spinach to wilt for a couple of minutes, then stir well.

6. As soon as the spinach has collapsed, add the yogurt mixture to the pan and cook, stirring until it just starts to bubble, then remove from the heat. Serve hot.

\\ Use this flavour bomb:
- Spooned over a bowl of Cauliflower Couscous (page 118; 42 cals) or shirataki noodles (calories negligible; page 116). Top with freshly grated Parmesan cheese if desired (44 cals for 10g/2tbsp).
- Spooned over a small jacket potato or sweet potato, adding a dollop of low-fat cottage cheese (88 cals for 100g) or a hard-boiled egg (74 cals) for extra protein.
- On top of a poached egg or two, or as a filling for a One-Egg Omelette (page 126).

\\ Keep in an airtight container in the fridge for up to 3 days. Reheat in the microwave. Stir very thoroughly: the sauce might curdle slightly on reheating at first, but stirring should emulsify it, and it is still delicious. Can also be frozen; reheat from frozen in the microwave.

CARAMELIZED ARTICHOKES

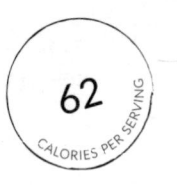

62 CALORIES PER SERVING

Gluten-free \\ Dairy-free \\ Vegan
NUTRITIONAL INFO PER SERVING: 3g fat, of which 0.2g saturates
7g carbohydrate, of which 2g sugars \\ 2g protein \\ 0.5g salt \\ 2g fibre

Canned artichoke hearts are a convenient fast-day treat, tasting way more indulgent than their mere 30 cals per 100g. Here's a simple treatment that makes them even yummier, concentrating their unique natural sweetness, imparting a meaty texture, and making them sing with garlic and chilli.

PREP & COOK TIME: **35 MINUTES**
SERVINGS: **2 LARGE**

1 x 400g can whole artichoke hearts in brine, drained
2 tsp extra-virgin rapeseed oil or sunflower oil

2 garlic cloves, crushed, or 1 tsp garlic powder or granules
½ tsp chilli flakes or powder, or to taste
large pinch of sea salt

1. Preheat the oven to 200°C/400°F/Gas Mark 6. Line a baking sheet with non-stick baking parchment.

2. Cut the artichoke hearts into quarters. Place in a bowl with the oil, garlic, chilli and salt, and toss gently but thoroughly with a rubber spatula to coat the artichokes well.

3. Transfer to the baking sheet and spread out in a single layer. Use the rubber spatula to scrape every last drop of dressing over the artichokes.

4   Bake for 30 minutes, until slightly crisp and patched with gold. Eat
hot, warm or cold.

\\ Use this flavour bomb:
- As a filling for a One-Egg Omelette (page 126) or to top scrambled eggs.
- Alongside a small jacket potato dressed with low-fat yogurt or cottage cheese.
- With a mixed-leaf and tomato salad seasoned with salt and balsamic vinegar; add a scoop of cottage cheese or a boiled egg for protein.

\\ Keep in an airtight container in the fridge for up to 3 days. Not suitable for freezing.

MEATY TOFU MINI-FILLETS

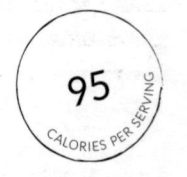

95 CALORIES PER SERVING

Gluten-free (if gluten-free soy sauce is used) \\ Dairy-free \\ Vegan
NUTRITIONAL INFO PER SERVING: 4g fat, of which 0.5g saturates
3g carbohydrate, of which 2g sugars \\ 9g protein \\ 3g salt \\ 0.9g fibre

Slow-roasting the marinated tofu strips gives them a toothsome, meaty
texture and concentrated flavour – a tasty protein-packed element to be
added to salads, noodles and vegetables.

PREP & COOK TIME: **5 MINUTES, PLUS 1
HOUR IN THE OVEN**
SERVINGS: **2 LARGE**

200g/7oz fresh firm tofu

spray oil
2 tbsp dark soy sauce
2 tbsp sweet cooking wine (page 36)
1 tsp seasoned rice vinegar
  or sushi vinegar

1   Preheat the oven to 120°C/250°F/Gas Mark ½.

2 | Pat the tofu dry with paper towels, then slice thinly into strips or rectangles, roughly 3mm/⅛in thick.

3 | Line a roasting pan with non-stick baking parchment. Spray the paper 5 or 6 times with oil. Lay the tofu slices on the paper side by side, quite close together.

4 | In a small bowl, combine the soy sauce, wine and vinegar, and stir. Spoon carefully over the tofu slices, giving each piece a good coating.

5 | Cook for about 1 hour, until the sauce has been absorbed and the tofu is firm and shrunken.

6 | Eat hot, warm or cold.

\\ Use this flavour bomb:
- Served warm on top of a bowl of noodles and steamed veg.
- Added to a broth of vegetables; noodles optional.
- Added to any salad configuration for protein and flavour.

\\ Keep in an airtight container in the fridge for up to 3 days. Can also be frozen.

PIQUANT MARINADE FOR TOFU

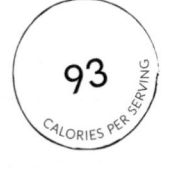

93
CALORIES PER SERVING

Gluten-free (if gluten-free soy sauce is used) \\ Dairy-free \\ Vegan
NUTRITIONAL INFO PER SERVING: 4g fat, of which 0.5g saturates
5g carbohydrate, of which 4g sugars \\ 9g protein \\ 3g salt \\ 1g fibre

Here we give plain old tofu a little bit of what it loves: salty soy sauce, chilli, sweet and sour vinegar, some ketchup for body, and time for all these folks to get acquainted, which really brings the tofu to life.

PREP & COOK TIME: **5 MINUTES, PLUS**
AT LEAST 1 HOUR MARINATING
SERVINGS: **2 LARGE**

200g/7oz fresh firm tofu

Marinade
2 tbsp teriyaki sauce or dark soy sauce
1 tsp hot chilli sauce
1 tbsp seasoned rice vinegar
  or sushi vinegar
1 tbsp ketchup

1. In a small bowl, whisk together the marinade ingredients until smooth.

2. Drain the tofu and wrap in paper towels to remove excess moisture. Cut into bite-sized cubes. Place in a container that will hold the cubes in one layer. Spoon the marinade over the tofu to coat evenly.

3. Cover and place in the fridge to marinate for at least 1 hour. Two hours is better, or overnight. Stir or shake gently once or twice while marinating, if possible.

4. Drain the excess marinade from the tofu (keep it: you can use it to season steamed vegetables to accompany the tofu) and eat cold or cook in one of the following ways:
   - microwave for 2 minutes
   - bake in a preheated oven at 220°C/425°F/Gas Mark 7 for 15 minutes
   - cook in a hot, ridged grill pan until striped with black on both sides.

\\ Use this flavour bomb:
   - Cold, with an Asian-style salad of crunchy salad leaves, fresh bean sprouts, cucumber slices, sugar snap peas, fresh coriander and pink pickled sushi ginger, all dressed with light soy sauce and fresh lime juice.
   - Hot, on a bed of noodles or Cauliflower Couscous (page 118) with added steamed veg.
   - Add some of the marinade to vegetables for microwave cooking, adding the marinated tofu to the cooking container to steam with the veg.

\\ Keep the tofu in its marinade container the fridge for up to 3 days. Can also be frozen, which alters the texture of the tofu to make it quite meaty; serve hot, reheated in the microwave from frozen or thawed.

SMOKY BBQ MARINADE FOR TOFU

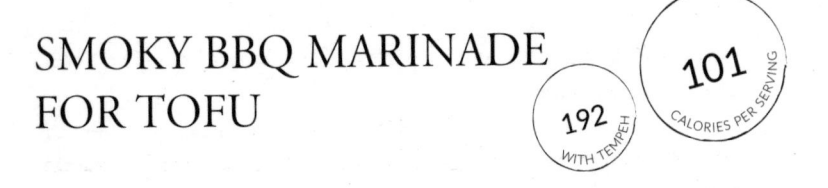

192 WITH TEMPEH

101 CALORIES PER SERVING

Gluten-free (if gluten-free soy sauce is used) \\ Dairy-free \\ Vegan
NUTRITIONAL INFO PER SERVING: (with tofu) 4g fat, of which 0.5g saturates
6g carbohydrate, of which 6g sugars \\ 9g protein \\ 2.9g salt \\ 3g fibre
(with tempeh) 7g fat, of which trace saturates
12g carbohydrate, of which 7g sugars \\ 22g protein \\ 2.9g salt \\ 6g fibre

Here, the classic sweet and tangy barbecue flavour gets its smokiness from Spanish smoked paprika. This can also be used for marinating tempeh (page 144).

PREP & COOK TIME: **5 MINUTES, PLUS
AT LEAST 1 HOUR MARINATING**
SERVINGS: **2 LARGE**

200g/7oz fresh firm tofu

Marinade
1 tbsp tomato purée (tomato paste)
1 tsp agave nectar or honey
2 tbsp dark soy sauce

1 tbsp cider vinegar
½ tsp English mustard
1 tsp smoked paprika (pimentón)
  or regular paprika
½ tsp ground cumin
½ tsp garlic powder or granules
large pinch of cayenne pepper,
  or to taste
1 tbsp water

1 Whisk together the marinade ingredients until smooth.

2   Drain the tofu and wrap in paper towels to remove excess moisture. Cut into 4 slabs about 1cm/½in thick. Choose a container that will hold the slabs in one layer. Spoon a little of the marinade into the container, then lay the tofu on top. Spoon the remaining marinade over it to coat evenly.

3   Cover and place in the fridge to marinate for at least 1 hour. Two hours is better, or overnight.

4   Lift the tofu from the excess marinade (keep it: you can use it to season steamed vegetables to accompany the tofu) and cook in one of the following ways:
- microwave for 2 minutes
- cook in a hot, ridged grill pan until striped with black on both sides
- bake on non-stick baking parchment in a preheated oven at 220°C/425°F/Gas Mark 7 for 15 minutes.

\\ Use this flavour bomb:
- Alongside a small jacket potato or Crushed Potatoes (page 125) and salad, or with salad alone.
- With a bowl of steamed vegetables and low-fat or shirataki noodles (page 116) seasoned with soy sauce and fresh lemon juice.
- The marinade can also be used to flavour vegetables before roasting in the oven.

\\ Keep the tofu in its marinade container in the fridge for up to 3 days. Can also be frozen, which alters the texture of the tofu to make it quite meaty – serve hot, reheated in the microwave from frozen or thawed.

ROASTED TEMPEH WITH CRISP CAPERS

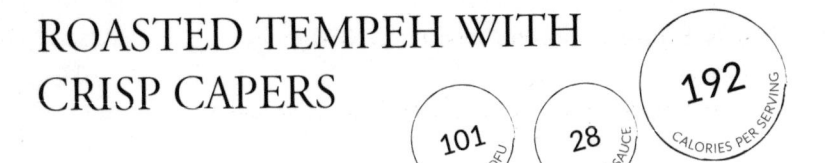

101 WITH TOFU

28 JUST THE SAUCE

192 CALORIES PER SERVING

Gluten-free (if gluten-free soy sauce is used) \\ Dairy-free \\ Vegan

NUTRITIONAL INFO PER SERVING: (with tempeh) 8g fat, of which 0.2g saturates 9g carbohydrate, of which 4g sugars \\ 21g protein \\ 1.6g salt \\ 6g fibre (with tofu) 6g fat, of which 0.7g saturates \\ 4g carbohydrate, of which 3g sugars \\ 91g protein \\ 1.6g salt \\ 0.9g fibre (sauce only) 2g fat, of which 0.2g saturates 3g carbohydrate, of which 3g sugars \\ 0.4g protein \\ 1.5g salt \\ 0g fibre

If you are not familiar with tempeh, you are in for a discovery. These cakes of fermented soybeans, originating in Indonesia, are much loved throughout Asia. Tempeh is available in health food shops, usually frozen, and usually in 200g packs, ideal for 2 servings. It doesn't score very highly in the glamour stakes, looking like a cake of compressed peanuts, sometimes encased in a web-like fuzz – this comes from the culture it is injected with. It does, however, take prizes for flavour and nutrition: it's nutty and chewy, and is packed with complete protein and many valuable nutrients, and weighs in at 150 cals per 100g. Traditionally it is pan-fried, but here's a scrumptious 5:2-friendly version. Build it into a meal with the suggestions below.

The uncooked sauce is lovely in itself and can be used as a punchy dressing for salad and steamed veg. Tofu also works really well in this recipe and can be substituted for the tempeh.

PREP & COOK TIME: **40 MINUTES**
SERVINGS: **2 LARGE**

200g/7oz tempeh
1 tbsp teriyaki sauce or dark soy sauce
1 tsp fresh lime juice

1 tsp English mustard
1 tsp agave nectar or honey
¼ tsp garlic powder or granules
½ tsp chilli flakes, or to taste
1 tsp olive or sunflower oil
2 tbsp capers in vinegar, drained

1 Preheat the oven to 200°C/400°F/Gas Mark 6.

2 Line a baking dish with non-stick baking parchment.

3 Cut the tempeh into about 10 long, thin slices, 1cm/½in thick.

4 In a small bowl, whisk together the remaining ingredients with a fork.

5 Dip each tempeh slice in the sauce (pushing the capers aside) and lay on the baking dish.

6 Spoon the remaining sauce, with capers, evenly over the tempeh.

7 Bake for 30 minutes, until the capers are crisp and the tempeh is deep golden.

\\ Use this flavour bomb:

- On top of a bowl of steamed vegetables and noodles (page 116), seasoned lightly with soy sauce and fresh lime juice.
- With Cauliflower Couscous (page 118) and steamed veg.
- With a salad of crisp leaves, cucumbers, spring onions and sliced palm hearts.

GREEN LIGHTNING SALSA

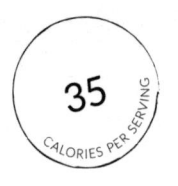

35

CALORIES PER SERVING

Gluten-free \\ Dairy-free \\ Vegan

NUTRITIONAL INFO PER SERVING: 3g fat. of which 0.3g saturates

2g carbohydrate, of which 2g sugars \\ 1g protein \\ trace salt \\ 0.2g fibre

Fresh coriander forms the base of this bright-green, flavour-packed sauce spiked with garlic and chilli and enriched with nutritious walnuts. Even if you are not a fan of coriander, you may find you love this sauce – the added flavours whizzed together transform the dominant herb. Remember to use the stems of the herb as well as the leaves: they are intensely flavourful.

PREP & COOK TIME: **10 MINUTES**
SERVINGS: **4 MEDIUM**

1 garlic clove
50g/1¾oz fresh coriander (cilantro),
  leaves and stems (weigh before
  washing, but do wash thoroughly
  and shake off excess water)

15g/½oz/2 tbsp walnuts
¼ tsp chilli flakes, or to taste
1 tsp agave nectar or honey
2 tbsp cider vinegar
  or red wine vinegar
sea salt to taste
3–4 tbsp water

1 | Peel the garlic and remove any sprout, then place in the blender and whizz until roughly chopped.

2 | Roughly chop the coriander and add to the blender along with everything else and purée, adding the water little by little to get the blades moving, but avoid watering it down too much.

3 | Let the motor run for 3 or 4 minutes and scrape down the sides from time to time, to be sure the sauce is completely smooth.

\\ Use this flavour bomb:

- With shirataki noodles: prepare according to instructions on page 116. Drain the noodles and toss with a little soy sauce. Stir through 1 chopped spring onion and 50g sliced sugar snap peas. Scrape into a bowl and top with 2–3 tbsp of the salsa.
- Spooned over a small jacket potato dressed with a dollop of low-fat yogurt or cottage cheese.
- As a dressing for a salad of mixed greens, artichoke hearts and hard-boiled egg.
- As a dip for celery, sugar snap peas, raw broccoli and cauliflower.

\\ Keep in an airtight container in the fridge for up to 3 days. Alternatively, pour into an ice-cube tray and pop out cubes as you need them – thaw a couple at a time at room temperature or in the microwave.

ONION CEVICHE

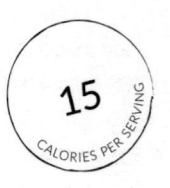

15

CALORIES PER SERVING

Gluten-free \\ Dairy-free \\ Vegan
NUTRITIONAL INFO PER SERVING: 0.1g fat, of which 0g saturates
3g carbohydrate, of which 3g sugars \\ 0.4g protein \\ 0.6g salt \\ 0.5g fibre

Here's a punchy little condiment; the raw onion softens and turns sweet and mild in its salty lemon-chilli bath. The resulting relish can be used in many ways – though my favourite is spooned over a sweet potato baked in its skin.

PREP & COOK TIME: **5 MINUTES,**
PLUS 30 MINUTES STANDING
SERVINGS: **2 MEDIUM**

50g/1¾oz/1 small white or red onion
¼ tsp fine salt
½ tsp chilli flakes
2 tbsp fresh lemon juice
pinch of sugar

1   Peel and finely chop the onion and place in a bowl.

2   Stir in the remaining ingredients and mix well.

3   Cover the bowl and leave to develop for about 30 minutes at room
temperature, then serve.

\\ Use this flavour bomb:
- Spooned over the mashed flesh of a sweet potato baked in its skin, with a
  side of cottage cheese or hard-boiled egg and some crunchy salad leaves.
- Tossed through cooled Cauliflower Couscous (page 118). Add steamed
  veg, or chopped spring onions and chopped tomatoes, plus a small handful
  of walnuts (95 cals for 15g/2 tbsp) and/or 1 tablespoon of low-fat yogurt
  (27 cals).
- Spread a low-cal wrap thinly with refried beans and warm in the oven or
  microwave. Lay thinly sliced tomato over the surface and spoon over the
  ceviche. Roll up and enjoy.

\\ Keep in an airtight container in the fridge for up to 3 days. Not suitable
for freezing.

EGG & PARMESAN DRESSING

98 CALORIES PER SERVING (20 PER TBSP)

Gluten-free

NUTRITIONAL INFO PER SERVING: (5 tbsp serving) 7g fat, of which 2g saturates
0.3g carbohydrate, of which 0.3g sugars \\ 8g protein \\ 0.3g salt \\ 0.1g fibre
(per tbsp) 1g fat, of which 0.5g saturates \\ 0.1g carbohydrate, of which
0.1g sugars \\ 2g protein \\ 0.1g salt \\ trace fibre

Here's a creamy, tangy, protein-packed Caesar-style dressing or sauce, which lends itself perfectly to a plate of crunchy leaves and veggies, providing a generous dose of nutrition and flavour with few calories. It's also delish with cooked spinach, mushrooms and potatoes, or as a dip for crudités.

PREP & COOK TIME: **12 MINUTES**
SERVINGS: **2 LARGE**

2 eggs
10g/¼oz Parmesan cheese
1 spring onion (scallion)

¼ tsp garlic powder or granules
　(optional)
1½ tbsp white wine vinegar
3 tbsp water
sea salt and freshly ground
　black pepper

1 Place the eggs in a small saucepan and cover with cold water. Bring to the boil and cook for 7 minutes, then drain and rinse under cold water until cool.

2 Meanwhile, grate the Parmesan and slice the spring onion.

3 Peel the eggs and place in the blender. Add the remaining ingredients and whizz at high speed until completely smooth and creamy. Serve.

\\ Use this flavour bomb:
- To make a Caesar-esque salad: arrange some crunchy romaine lettuce or

Little Gem hearts on a plate. Break up a couple of melba toasts (ideally wholegrain) and scatter over the leaves as croutons, then top with the dressing. Finish with extra grated Parmesan (22 cals per tbsp).

- Dribbled over a grilled mushroom, wilted spinach and a Perfect Poached Egg (page 133), as shown on the cover.
- In a bowl surrounded with crunchy crudités such as celery, pepper strips, raw broccoli and cauliflower, and boiled baby potatoes.

\\ Keep in an airtight container in the fridge for up to 3 days. Can also be frozen.

MAGIC ASIAN DRESSING

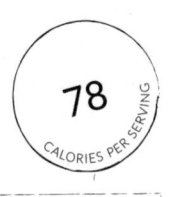

78 CALORIES PER SERVING

Gluten-free (if gluten-free soy sauce is used) \\ Dairy-free \\ Vegan
NUTRITIONAL INFO PER SERVING: (2 tbsp serving) 0g fat, of which 0g saturates
18g carbohydrate, of which 18g sugars \\ 1g protein \\ 4g salt \\ 0.6g fibre

You can't beat the high-impact flavour of a well-balanced Asian quartet of sweet, sour, salty and hot. A little finely grated carrot in the mix carries the tune and gives a toothsome texture to this versatile dressing.

PREP & COOK TIME: **5 MINUTES**
SERVINGS: **4 LARGE**

1 garlic clove
3 tbsp fresh lime juice

3 tbsp light soy sauce
2 tbsp agave nectar or honey
¼–½ tsp chilli flakes, or to taste
freshly ground black pepper
25g/1oz carrot

1 Peel the garlic and remove any sprout, then crush into a small bowl.

2   Add the lime juice, soy sauce, agave or honey, chilli and pepper.

3   Peel the carrot and grate finely, then stir into the sauce, combining thoroughly.

4   The sauce can be used immediately, but becomes hotter and more flavourful if left to infuse for a few minutes or hours.

\\ Use this flavour bomb:

- With any combination of steamed veg, tofu and/or noodles, served hot, or cold as a salad. Lovely with steamed or raw bean sprouts.
- To marinate tofu for an hour or more, or simply use as a dressing or cooking liquid for the tofu.
- With Cauliflower Couscous (page 118) or wholegrain rice, plus tofu or boiled egg for protein and your vegetables of choice.
- Drizzled over a mixed-leaf salad with hard-boiled eggs.

\\ Keep in an airtight container in the fridge for up to 3 days. Not suitable for freezing.

NAPOLI SAUCE

43
CALORIES PER SERVING

Gluten-free \\ Dairy-free \\ Vegan
NUTRITIONAL INFO PER SERVING: 2g fat, of which 0.2g saturates
6g carbohydrate, of which 5g sugars \\ 2g protein \\ 0.1g salt \\ 1g fibre

The classic Italian tomato sauce gets a low-cal makeover but tastes just as satisfying. Slather this over shirataki noodles (page 116) or Cauliflower Couscous (page 118), or make a fast-day pizza (see below).

PREP & COOK TIME: **20 MINUTES**
SERVINGS: **2 LARGE**

2 spring onions (scallions)
2 garlic cloves
1 tsp olive oil
250ml/9fl oz/generous 1 cup tomato
  passata (strained tomatoes)

1 tsp balsamic vinegar
½ tsp agave nectar or honey
¼ tsp mixed dried herbs
sea salt and freshly ground
  black pepper
handful of fresh basil leaves (optional)

1 | Chop the spring onions and crush the garlic.

2 | Heat a saucepan or frying pan over a low heat and add the oil. Add the onions and garlic, and cook for about 2 minutes, until fragrant.

3 | Add the passata, vinegar, agave or honey, dried herbs and seasoning. Bring to the boil, then reduce the heat and simmer, stirring occasionally, for 15 minutes, until thickened.

4 | Tear the fresh basil (if using) into the sauce and serve with desired accompaniments.

\\ Use this flavour bomb:

- Spooned over a bowl of Cauliflower Couscous (page 118) or noodles (page 116). Top with freshly grated Parmesan cheese if desired (44 cals for 10g/2 tbsp).
- Spread over a low-cal wrap, top with reduced-fat grated mozzarella, then bake at 200°C/400°F/Gas Mark 6 for about 7 minutes until bubbly. Eat as a pizza or roll up and slice in half.
- Spooned over a small jacket potato or sweet potato, adding a dollop of low-fat cottage cheese (44 cals for 50g) or a hard-boiled egg (74 cals) for extra protein.
- On top of a poached egg or two, or as a filling for a One-Egg Omelette (page 126).

\\ Keep in an airtight container in the fridge for up to 3 days. Can also be frozen.

PUTTANESCA SAUCE

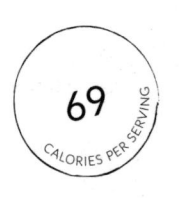

69
CALORIES PER SERVING

Gluten-free \\ Dairy-free \\ Vegan
NUTRITIONAL INFO PER SERVING: 3g fat, of which 0.5g saturates
8g carbohydrate, of which 3g sugars \\ 2g protein \\ 1.2g salt \\ 4g fibre

A classic Italian sauce, traditionally used for making *spaghetti alla puttanesca*, or 'whore's pasta', so called because of its spicy, fleshy nature – it's bursting with flavour and substance.

PREP. & COOK TIME: **30 MINUTES**
SERVINGS: **2 LARGE**

2 spring onions (scallions)
2 garlic cloves
50g/1¾oz/about ½ red pepper
1 tsp olive oil
250ml/9fl oz/generous 1 cup tomato passata (strained tomatoes)
1 tsp balsamic vinegar

½ tsp agave nectar or honey
¼ tsp mixed dried herbs
2 tsp drained capers in vinegar
25g/1oz drained green or black olives in brine
½ tsp chilli flakes, or to taste
sea salt and freshly ground black pepper
handful of fresh basil leaves (optional)

1 Chop the spring onions, crush the garlic and roughly chop the red pepper.

2 Heat a saucepan or frying pan over a low heat and add the oil. Add the onions, garlic and red pepper, and cook for about 2 minutes, until fragrant.

3 | Add the passata, vinegar, agave or honey, dried herbs, capers, olives, chilli flakes and seasoning. Bring to the boil, then reduce the heat and simmer, stirring occasionally, for 15 minutes, until thickened.

4 | Tear the fresh basil (if using) into the sauce, stir and serve with desired accompaniments.

\\ Use this flavour bomb:
- Spooned over a bowl of Cauliflower Couscous (page 118) or noodles (page 116). Top with freshly grated Parmesan cheese if desired (44 cals for 10g/ 2 tbsp).
- Spread over a low-cal wrap, top with reduced-fat mozzarella, then bake at 200°C/400°F/Gas Mark 6 for about 7 minutes until bubbly. Eat as a pizza or roll up and slice in half.
- Spooned over a small jacket potato or sweet potato, adding a dollop of low-fat cottage cheese (44 cals for 50g) or a hard-boiled egg (74 cals) for extra protein.
- On top of a poached egg or two, or as a filling for a One-Egg Omelette (page 126).

\\ Keep in an airtight container in the fridge for up to 3 days. Can also be frozen.

ALMOND & TOMATO SAUCE

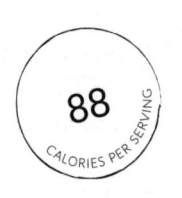

88 CALORIES PER SERVING

Gluten-free \\ Dairy-free \\ Vegan
NUTRITIONAL INFO PER SERVING: (4 tbsp) 7g fat, of which 0.6g saturates
2g carbohydrate, of which 2g sugars \\ 4g protein \\ 0.1g salt \\ 0.5g fibre

In this stripped-down version of the classic *salsa romesco* from Catalonia in Spain, a handful of ingredients combine to dazzling effect. This is one of my all-time favourites for dipping or dressing veg and salad, and it is also wonderful with eggs, potatoes and even noodles (see suggestions below).

PREP & COOK TIME: **10 MINUTES**
SERVINGS: **2 LARGE**

25g/1oz flaked almonds
1 garlic clove
100g/3½oz canned chopped tomatoes
  with juice

2 tsp red wine vinegar
3 tbsp water
sea salt and freshly ground
  black pepper
cayenne pepper (optional)

1 Heat a frying pan over a medium–high heat and add the almonds. Toast in the pan, stirring frequently, until golden, about 2–3 minutes, then remove the almonds to a plate to cool. (Alternatively, toast on a baking sheet in an oven preheated to 200°C/400°F/Gas Mark 6, until golden.)

2 Meanwhile, peel the garlic and remove any sprout.

3 Put the garlic in the blender and whizz until finely chopped.

4 | Add the remaining ingredients, including the cooled almonds, and whizz at high speed until completely smooth. Taste for seasoning and serve.

\\ Use this flavour bomb:

- As a dip for crudités, with or without boiled new potatoes.
- As a sauce for a simple omelette or poached or scrambled eggs.
- Heated in the microwave and drizzled over a small baked potato, sweet potato or Crushed Potatoes (page 125), with cottage cheese or yogurt. Accompany with a mixed-leaf and tomato salad.
- Stirred through noodles, or stir-fried with noodles for a couple of minutes. Top with freshly grated Parmesan (22 cals per tbsp).

\\ Keep in an airtight container in the fridge for up to 3 days. Can also be frozen; thaw thoroughly at room temperature.

CREAMY SESAME SAUCE

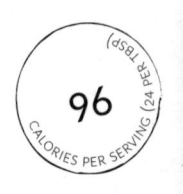

96 CALORIES PER SERVING (24 PER TBSP)

Gluten-free (if gluten-free soy sauce is used)
NUTRITIONAL INFO PER SERVING: (4 tbsp serving) 6g fat, of which 1g saturates
4g carbohydrate, of which 4g sugars \\ 5g protein \\ 1.4g salt \\ 1g fibre

Three ingredients here add up to much more than the sum of their parts. If you have some ready-toasted sesame seeds in your cupboard (see page 37), this takes 1 minute to throw together. This is quite a salty mixture from the dark soy, which makes it perfect as a punchy dip for unseasoned raw crudités, or spooned over a naked salad. Reduce the soy sauce quantity for a softer flavour.

PREP & COOK TIME: **30 MINUTES**
SERVINGS: **2 LARGE**

2 tbsp sesame seeds
100g/3½oz/scant ½ cup low-fat yogurt
1 tbsp dark soy sauce

1   Heat a frying pan over a medium–high heat and add the sesame seeds. Cook, stirring frequently, until golden and popping, about 3–4 minutes, then remove to a plate to cool completely.

2   Measure the yogurt into a small bowl. Stir in the cooled sesame seeds and soy sauce, then serve.

\\ Use this flavour bomb:

- As a dip for crudités, with or without boiled new potatoes.
- As a sauce for a simple omelette or poached or scrambled eggs.
- Drizzled over a small baked potato, sweet potato or Crushed Potatoes (page 125). Accompany with a leafy salad.

\\ Keep in an airtight container in the fridge for up to 3 days, though fresh is best. Not suitable for freezing.

CHAPTER 6
SPEEDY BREAKFASTS

WHETHER OR NOT you want to start your fast day by breaking last night's fast is up to you. Most 5:2 fasters seem to either forgo breakfast altogether or keep it to a minimum so there's more to look forward to later in the day. However, a little bit of protein first thing will help you feel full for longer. If you're a busy person, breakfast is likely to be the meal you grab on the run or spend no more than a few minutes throwing together. This chapter is designed for you.

Most of the recipes in this chapter can also be enjoyed as a speedy lunch or dinner too.

5 ultra-quick breakfast ideas at 100 cals or less:

- Wholegrain rice cake with 50g low-fat cottage cheese and a light sprinkle of sesame seeds – about 70 cals

- 2 wholegrain melba toasts with 1 triangle of low-fat cheese spread – about 50 cals

- 50g low-fat yogurt with 50g blueberries and 1 tsp honey – about 100 cals

- A hard-boiled egg mashed with 1 small chopped tomato, 2 tsp low-fat yogurt, salt and pepper – about 100 cals

- 100g frozen peas or sweetcorn, cooked in the microwave, drained and mixed with 1 tbsp light cream cheese – about 100 cals

PERFECT PORRIDGE

There's a minor science to making perfect porridge; it's not something you can 'eyeball'. As a bit of a porridge fan (especially in the winter), over the years I've devised the ideal ratio of rolled oats to liquid: 25g to 170ml for one serving, cooked in the microwave. The easiest way to measure the liquid is in a 125ml (½-cup) measure, plus 3 tbsp. Call me pedantic, but in this case it's important.

Most of the time, I enjoy my porridge with a pat of butter and a slathering of honey or dark-brown sugar. For fast days, I've devised these slimmer versions. I always use soy milk as I think it gives the creamiest flavour, but you could use semi-skimmed milk instead.

APPLE CINNAMON PORRIDGE

Dairy-free \\ Vegan
NUTRITIONAL INFO PER SERVING: 3g fat, of which 0.1g saturates
23g carbohydrate, of which 6g sugars \\ 5g protein \\ 0.1g salt \\ 3g fibre

PREP & COOK TIME: **6 MINUTES**
SERVINGS: **1 MEDIUM**

25g/1oz/¹⁄₃ cup rolled oats
125ml/4fl oz/½ cup measured
  half cloudy apple juice + half
  unsweetened soy milk

3 tbsp water
1 tsp ultra-low-calorie sugar substitute
  (or to taste)
large pinch of ground cinnamon
pinch of salt

1 Choose a microwave-safe serving bowl. Pop it on the scales and measure in your oats.

2 Add all the remaining ingredients and stir.

3 Cover and microwave on high power for 2 minutes.

4 Remove from the microwave (carefully, as it will be very hot), stir, cover and stand for 1 minute, then serve.

CINNAMON ALMOND PORRIDGE

117 CALORIES PER SERVING

Dairy-free \\ Vegan

NUTRITIONAL INFO PER SERVING: 3g fat, of which 0.1g saturates
17g carbohydrate, of which 0.1g sugars \\ 5g protein \\ 0.1g salt \\ 3g fibre

PREP & COOK TIME: **6 MINUTES**
SERVINGS: **1 MEDIUM**

25g/1oz/⅓ cup rolled oats
125ml/4fl oz/½ cup measured half
  unsweetened soy milk + half water

3 tbsp water
1 tsp ultra-low-calorie sugar substitute
  (or to taste)
large pinch of ground cinnamon
1 or 2 drops pure almond extract
pinch of salt

Prepare as for Apple Cinnamon Porridge.

STRAWBERRY VANILLA PORRIDGE

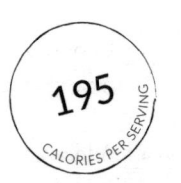

195
CALORIES PER SERVING

Dairy-free \\ Vegan
NUTRITIONAL INFO PER SERVING: 3g fat, of which 0.1g saturates
36g carbohydrate, of which 19g sugars \\ 5g protein \\ 0.1g salt \\ 3g fibre

Any flavour jam can be substituted for strawberry.

PREP & COOK TIME: 6 MINUTES
SERVINGS: **1 MEDIUM**

25g/1oz/⅓ cup rolled oats
125ml/4fl oz/½ cup measured half
  unsweetened soy milk + half water

3 tbsp water
2 or 3 drops pure vanilla extract
pinch of salt
1 tbsp low-sugar strawberry jam

Prepare as for Apple Cinnamon Porridge, adding the jam after step 4. Don't stir the strawberry jam completely through the mixture – leave it to create a slightly marbled effect.

SMOOTHIES

Smoothies are a breakfast staple, but when made with lots of fruit can be surprisingly high in calories. By using xanthan gum, you can thicken just about any liquid in the blender to a smoothie consistency, adding minimal calories. Xanthan gum is found in many processed foods as an emulsifier. Although it is created in a laboratory, it is a sugar derived from bacteria and is usually packaged for home use by natural food companies who recommend it for making gluten-free bread, so it's available, as a powder, in health food shops and some supermarkets. It's a good source of dietary fibre.

Note: A scoop of protein powder (about 70 cals) can be added to all of the following for increased nutrition and appetite suppression.

CHOCOLATE VELVET SMOOTHIE

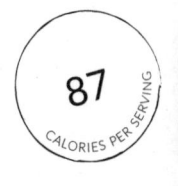

Gluten-free

NUTRITIONAL INFO PER SERVING: 5g fat, of which 1g saturates
2g carbohydrate, of which 0.5g sugars \\ 8g protein \\ 0.3g salt \\ 2g fibre

PREP & COOK TIME: **3 MINUTES**
SERVINGS: **1 LARGE**

250ml/9fl oz/generous 1 cup
  unsweetened soy milk or skimmed
  (non-fat) milk

1 tbsp unsweetened cocoa
1 tbsp ultra-low-calorie sugar
  substitute (or to taste)
pinch of ground cinnamon
  or freshly grated nutmeg (optional)
¼ tsp xanthan gum

Place everything in a blender and whizz for 1 minute, until thick.

BANANA ALMOND SMOOTHIE

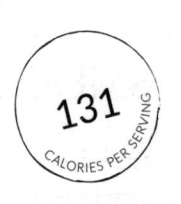
131
CALORIES PER SERVING

Gluten-free

NUTRITIONAL INFO PER SERVING: 2g fat, of which 0.4g saturates

23g carbohydrate, of which 21g sugars \\ 5g protein \\ 0.1g salt \\ 2g fibre

PREP & COOK TIME: **3 MINUTES**

SERVINGS: **1 LARGE**

1 small banana

125ml/4fl oz/½ cup unsweetened soy milk or skimmed (non-fat) milk

125ml/4fl oz/½ cup cold water

1 tbsp ultra-low-calorie sugar substitute (or to taste)

¼ tsp pure almond extract

¼ tsp ground cinnamon

¼ tsp xanthan gum

1 Peel the banana, break into 3 or 4 pieces, and place in a blender.

2 Add everything else to the blender and whizz for 1 minute, until thick.

MANGO & GINGER FRAPPÉ

123
CALORIES PER SERVING

Gluten-free

NUTRITIONAL INFO PER SERVING: 2g fat, of which 0.4g saturates
21g carbohydrate, of which 20g sugars \\ 4g protein \\ 0.1g salt \\ 6g fibre

PREP & COOK TIME: **5 MINUTES**
SERVINGS: **1 LARGE**

1cm/½in piece fresh ginger
150g/5½oz fresh mango, peeled
125ml/4fl oz/½ cup unsweetened soy
  milk or skimmed (non-fat) milk

125ml/4fl oz/½ cup water
squeeze of fresh lime juice
1 tbsp ultra-low-calorie sugar
  substitute (or to taste)
¼ tsp xanthan gum
5 large ice cubes

1   Peel and grate the ginger and cut the mango into chunks.

2   Place everything in a blender and whizz for 2 minutes, until the ice is puréed.

ICED MOCHA FRAPPÉ

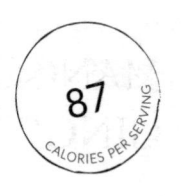

87 CALORIES PER SERVING

Gluten-free

NUTRITIONAL INFO PER SERVING: 5g fat, of which 1g saturates
2g carbohydrate, of which 0.5g sugars \\ 8g protein \\ 0.3g salt \\ 2g fibre

PREP & COOK TIME: **3 MINUTES**
SERVINGS: **1 LARGE**

250ml/9fl oz/generous 1 cup
 unsweetened soy milk or skimmed
 (non-fat) milk

1 tbsp unsweetened cocoa
2 tsp instant coffee powder
1 tbsp ultra-low-calorie sugar
 substitute (or to taste)
¼ tsp xanthan gum
5 large ice cubes

Place everything in a blender and whizz for 2 minutes, until the ice
is puréed.

BREAKFAST MISO CUP

78
CALORIES PER SERVING

Gluten-free (if gluten-free miso and soy sauce are used) \\ Dairy-free \\ Vegan
NUTRITIONAL INFO PER SERVING: 3g fat, of which 0.3g saturates
5g carbohydrate, of which 0.4g sugars \\ 7g protein \\ 1.9g salt \\ 0.2g fibre

---

Miso soup is common breakfast fare in Japan – nourishing, warming and delicious. I often add a handful of frozen tofu cubes to my morning miso. If using frozen tofu (page 31), just pour boiling water over it, leave until thawed, then drain and use in the recipe. Any type of miso can be used for this, though a mild white miso is best (page 32). You can also use instant miso soup.

PREP & COOK TIME: **5 MINUTES**
SERVINGS: **1 MEDIUM**

½ spring onion (scallion)
50g/1¾oz tofu, firm or silken
25g/1oz/1 heaped tbsp miso paste

Optional seasonings
squeeze of fresh lemon or lime juice
a few drops of soy sauce
cayenne pepper

1. Boil a small amount of water in the kettle. Meanwhile, slice the spring onion and cut the tofu into small cubes. Once boiled, leave the water to settle and cool for a minute or two.

2. Measure the miso into a mug. Pour a splash of hot water over it and stir to dissolve the miso. (Using hot but not boiling water maintains the optimum nutrition in the miso and prevents it from curdling.)

3. Stir in the spring onion and tofu. Re-boil the kettle.

4. Top up with about 125ml/4fl oz/½ cup boiling water, stir, and add your optional seasonings to taste.

CREAMY MUSHROOM CAPS

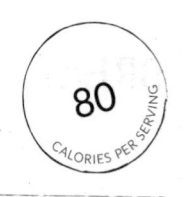

80 CALORIES PER SERVING

Gluten-free

NUTRITIONAL INFO PER SERVING: 6g fat, of which 2g saturates

1g carbohydrate, of which 1g sugars \\ 6g protein \\ 0.3g salt \\ 1g fibre

---

A morning microwave miracle, all done in less than 5 minutes. Mushrooms are so full of tasty juice, they lend themselves perfectly to microwave cooking, and here the juices mingle with cream cheese and herbs to form a rich sauce that is great on toast (69 cals for an average 30g slice of wholemeal bread; no butter necessary) or with poached egg (74 cals) or scrambled egg (99 cals).

PREP & COOK TIME: **4 MINUTES**
SERVINGS: **1 MEDIUM**

1 large flat mushroom (about 75g/2¾oz with stem)
1 tsp extra-virgin rapeseed oil or olive oil

25g/1oz/about 1 heaped tbsp light cream cheese
large pinch of herbs: fresh basil, fresh or dried thyme, dill or mixed herbs
sea salt and freshly ground black pepper

1 Snap out the stem of the mushroom and lay the cap gill-side-up in a microwave-safe container. Drizzle the oil over the gills.

2 Spread the cream cheese inside the cap, then top with herbs and season with salt and pepper.

3 Cover and microwave on high power for 1 minute 30 seconds, then stand for 30 seconds (the mushroom should be slightly collapsed, soft and juicy, the sauce bubbly and mingling with the mushroom juice).

4 Transfer to a plate, spoon any stray sauce over, and enjoy.

DILL & GARLIC TOMATOES ON CHEESE TOAST

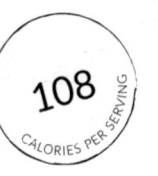

108 CALORIES PER SERVING

NUTRITIONAL INFO PER SERVING: 2g fat, of which 1g saturates
15g carbohydrate, of which 4g sugars \\ 6g protein \\ 0.6g salt \\ 4g fibre

Five minutes to a delicious breakfast. Thank you, microwave! This is one of my absolute faves and is great for lunch too. A poached egg could be substituted for the toast or added on top of the tomatoes. Of course, fresh crushed garlic and chopped fresh dill can be used instead of dried, but I'm saving time here, without losing flavour.

PREP & COOK TIME: **5 MINUTES**
SERVINGS: **1 LARGE**

100g/3½oz fresh ripe cherry tomatoes
½ tsp garlic powder or granules
½ tsp dried dill

torn fresh basil leaves (optional)
sea salt and freshly ground
   black pepper
1 slice of wholemeal toast
   (69 cals for 30g slice), spread with
   15g/½oz low-fat spreadable cheese

1 | Put the tomatoes in a small microwaveable container. Pierce each tomato with the tip of a small knife to prevent them exploding. Add the garlic, dill, basil (if using), and season with salt and pepper. Stir.

2 | Cover and microwave on high power for 1 minute, then stand for 1 minute. You should have a hot saucy mixture.

3 | Meanwhile, toast your bread and spread with cheese.

4 | Pour the tomato mixture on top of the toast and serve.

EGG IN A FRAME

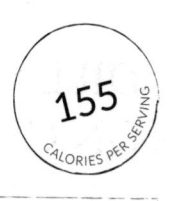

155 CALORIES PER SERVING

NUTRITIONAL INFO PER SERVING: 10g fat, of which 2g saturates
8g carbohydrate, of which 0.5g sugars \\ 8g protein \\ 0.5g salt \\ 1g fibre

This childhood favourite is perfect for fast days. You lose some of the calories from the bread to make room for an appetite-busting egg and need very little fat to make it delicious. The calorie count of bread varies, but you can get an accurate count from packaged bread by doing this: cut the hole out of the bread slice, then weigh the 'frame'. Put a decimal point in front of the gram weight (e.g. 24 grams, 0.24) and multiply by the cals per 100g on the label.

PREP & COOK TIME: **5 MINUTES**
SERVINGS: **1 MEDIUM**

1 slice of wholemeal bread

spray oil
1 tsp margarine
1 egg
sea salt and ground black pepper

1 Use a pastry cutter or the rim of a glass, about 7cm/3in in diameter, to cut a hole in the middle of the bread.

2 Heat a non-stick frying pan over a medium heat. Spray four times with spray oil and add the bread 'frame'.

3 Pop the margarine inside the hole in the bread until it melts, then break in the egg. Season. Once the bottom of the egg has set, flip the whole thing over and cook the other side. After a couple of minutes, the egg should be cooked to a soft consistency. Give it a poke with a sharp knife to make sure the egg white has cooked through. (If you prefer a well-done egg, keep flipping until set all the way through.)

SCRAMBLED EGGS & VARIATIONS

It has to be said that scrambled eggs are best when endowed with a generous pat of butter, and possibly even a spoonful of crème fraîche stirred in at the end. Alas, such luxurious eggs are not for fast days. However, a scrambled egg can still be a quick 5:2 breakfast solution, with or without a small slice of wholemeal toast.

How do you like your scrambled eggs? There seem to be two camps: fluffy or creamy. Both can be achieved with the techniques outlined here. I've also included some tasty additions that don't compromise speed or calories. All recipes are for one egg. Multiply accordingly, though cooking times may change. Your best non-stick frying pan is a must; a flexible spatula a bonus.

See also Omelettes (page 126) and Perfect Poached Eggs (page 133).

A FLUFFY SCRAMBLED EGG

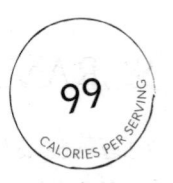

99 CALORIES PER SERVING

Gluten-free

NUTRITIONAL INFO PER SERVING: **8g** fat, of which **2g** saturates

0.7g carbohydrate, of which **0.7g** sugars \\ **7g** protein \\ **0.2g** salt \\ **0g** fibre

---

PREP & COOK TIME: **3 MINUTES**

SERVINGS: **1 MEDIUM**

1 egg

1 tbsp semi-skimmed (low-fat) milk

sea salt and freshly ground
  black pepper

½ tsp margarine or butter

1. Heat a non-stick frying pan over a medium–high heat.

2. Break the egg into a small bowl or teacup. Add the milk, salt and pepper, and use a fork to beat thoroughly.

3. Plop the margarine or butter into the hot frying pan and use a spatula to spread it over the surface.

4. Pour in the egg and swirl to coat the pan. The bottom should set immediately; fold from the edges, turning the cooked underside over the uncooked middle.

5. Continue folding, breaking it up slightly as you go to ensure even cooking. Remove from the heat when just set throughout and serve immediately.

A CREAMY SCRAMBLED EGG

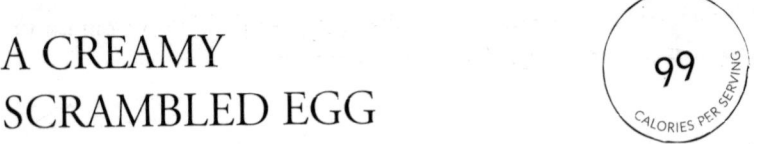

99 CALORIES PER SERVING

Gluten-free

NUTRITIONAL INFO PER SERVING: 8g fat, of which 2g saturates
0.7g carbohydrate, of which 0.7g sugars \\ 7g protein \\ 0.2g salt \\ 0g fibre

---

PREP & COOK TIME: **6 MINUTES**
SERVINGS: **1 MEDIUM**

1 egg
1 tbsp semi-skimmed (low-fat) milk
sea salt and freshly ground black
 pepper
½ tsp margarine or butter

1. Heat a non-stick frying pan over a low heat.

2. Break the egg into a small bowl or teacup. Add the milk, salt and pepper, and use a fork to beat thoroughly.

3. Plop the margarine or butter into the frying pan and use a spatula to spread it over the surface as it gradually melts.

4. Pour in the egg and swirl to coat the pan. Stir every 30 seconds or so for about 4 minutes, until set to your liking, and serve immediately.

The following techniques are for fluffy eggs (page 173) but you can use the technique for creamy eggs (opposite) if you prefer.

CHEESE & HERB SCRAMBLE

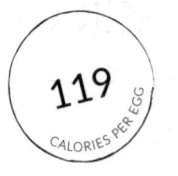

119 CALORIES PER EGG

Gluten-free

NUTRITIONAL INFO PER SERVING: 9g fat, of which 3g saturates

1g carbohydrate, of which 1g sugars \\ 8g protein \\ 0.6g salt \\ 0g fibre

---

PREP & COOK TIME: **4 MINUTES**
SERVINGS: **1 MEDIUM**

1 egg
15g/½oz (1 triangle) low-fat cheese
  spread

¼ tsp dried dill or mixed dried herbs
sea salt and freshly ground
  black pepper
½ tsp margarine or butter

1. Heat a non-stick frying pan over a medium–high heat.

2. Break the egg into a small bowl. Add the cheese and use a fork to beat thoroughly, pressing the cheese so it breaks up into lumps. Season with pepper and a pinch of salt (bearing in mind that the cheese is salty).

3. Plop the margarine or butter into the frying pan and use a spatula to spread it over the surface.

4. Pour in the egg mixture and swirl to coat the pan. The bottom should set immediately; fold from the edges, turning the cooked underside over the uncooked middle. Continue folding, breaking it up slightly as you go to ensure even cooking. Remove from the heat when just set throughout and serve immediately.

MEXICAN SCRAMBLE

130 CALORIES PER SERVING

Gluten-free

NUTRITIONAL INFO PER SERVING: 9g fat, of which 3g saturates

3g carbohydrate, of which 3g sugars \\ 9g protein \\ 0.6g salt \\ 0.9g fibre

PREP & COOK TIME: **4 MINUTES**
SERVINGS: **1 MEDIUM**

1 spring onion (scallion)
½ small green chilli (or a whole one if you dare!)
2 cherry tomatoes

1 egg
15g/½oz (1 triangle) low-fat cheese spread
sea salt and freshly ground black pepper
½ tsp margarine or butter
2 tsp Mexican salsa, to serve (optional)

1 Heat a non-stick frying pan over a medium–high heat.

2 Chop the spring onion and chilli. Slice or quarter the tomatoes.

3 Break the egg into a small bowl. Add the cheese and use a fork to beat thoroughly, pressing the cheese so it breaks up into lumps. Season with pepper and a pinch of salt (bearing in mind that the cheese is salty).

4 Plop the margarine or butter into the frying pan and use a spatula to spread it over the surface. Add the onion and chilli and stir.

5 Pour in the egg mixture and swirl to coat the pan. Add the tomatoes. The bottom should set immediately; fold from the edges, turning the cooked underside over the uncooked middle. Continue folding, breaking it up slightly as you go to ensure even cooking. Remove from the heat when just set throughout and serve immediately, topped with salsa, if desired.

PALM HEART SCRAMBLE

113 CALORIES PER SERVING

Gluten-free \\ Dairy-free
NUTRITIONAL INFO PER SERVING: 9g fat, of which 2g saturates
1g carbohydrate, of which 0g sugars \\ 7g protein \\ 0.3g salt \\ 0.6g fibre

---

Oh, blessed are canned palm hearts on fast days! Here's a dead simple and delectable breakfast or lunch or well, anytime, option - palm hearts scrambled with egg. You could add chopped spring onion or chilli, but I think the naked simplicity of just the egg and palm hearts cannot be improved upon. They have a remarkable affinity. I enjoy this with lots of freshly ground black pepper, and if the calorie ceiling allows, on a slice of wholegrain toast.

PREP & COOK TIME: **10 MINUTES**
SERVINGS: **1 LARGE**

25g/1oz palm hearts

1 tsp margarine or butter
1 egg
sea salt and freshly ground
   black pepper

1 Chop the palm hearts roughly.

2 Heat a non-stick frying pan over a low–medium heat. Add the margarine and, once melted, add the palm hearts and cook until lightly browned. Scrape to the middle of the pan.

3 Beat the egg with a little salt and pepper, and pour over the palm hearts. Allow the bottom to set, then stir, folding, until scrambled but not dry. Serve immediately.

SPEEDY FRITTATAS

These substantial open-faced omelettes add up to around half your fast-day calorie allowance. They could just as easily reside in the 'Easy Fast-Day Meals' chapter, as they can be enjoyed any time of day. Since they're all done in under 10 minutes, even the groggiest faster can rustle one up in the early hours to fuel up for the day. These are pretty generous portions, so you could divide a frittata in half and eat the other half later in the day, with salad or steamed veggies.

CREAMY CHILLI SWEETCORN FRITTATA

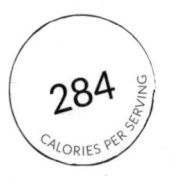

284 CALORIES PER SERVING

Gluten-free

NUTRITIONAL INFO PER SERVING: 15g fat, of which 4g saturates
19g carbohydrate, of which 3g sugars \\ 19g protein \\ 0.8g salt \\ 3g fibre

The American in me just adores the trio of cheese, corn and chilli, and a frittata is the ideal frame for this sublime flavour and texture combo. If your calorie ceiling allows, slather an extra portion of cheese spread on top of the finished item (25 extra calories).

PREP & COOK TIME: **8 MINUTES**
SERVINGS: **1 LARGE**

100g/3½oz frozen sweetcorn
15g/½oz (1 triangle) low-fat cheese
  spread

1 small red or green chilli
2 eggs
sea salt and freshly ground
  black pepper
spray oil

1. Place the sweetcorn in a microwave-safe container and cook on high power for 2 minutes, then drain and transfer to a small bowl.

2. Add the cheese to the hot corn and stir with a fork, letting it melt and break up into small lumps.

3. Use scissors to snip in the chilli and stir.

4. Add the eggs, salt and pepper, and whisk until well combined.

5. Heat a grillproof non-stick frying pan over a medium heat and spray 4 times with spray oil. Preheat the grill to high.

6. Pour the egg mixture into the pan and swirl to meet the edge of the pan.

7. Cook until the underside is light golden, about 2 minutes, then place the pan under the grill until the top is set, about 1–2 minutes, and serve.

ARTICHOKE, PARMESAN & BASIL FRITTATA

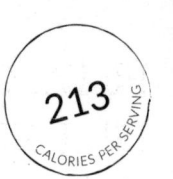

213
CALORIES PER SERVING

Gluten-free

NUTRITIONAL INFO PER SERVING: 14g fat, of which 5g saturates
5g carbohydrate, of which 1g sugars \\ 17g protein \\ 3.9g salt \\ 1.6g fibre

A classic Italian trio.

PREP & COOK TIME: **7 MINUTES**
SERVINGS: **1 LARGE**

85g/3oz (about 3 whole) canned
    artichoke hearts, drained
10g/¼oz Parmesan cheese

2 eggs
sea salt and freshly ground
    black pepper
spray oil
2 fresh basil tips

1 Slice the artichoke hearts and finely grate the Parmesan.

2 In a small bowl, beat the eggs, salt and pepper with a fork until
   well mixed.

3 Heat a grillproof non-stick frying pan over a medium heat and spray 4
   times with spray oil. Preheat the grill to high.

4 Pour the egg mixture into the pan and swirl to meet the edge of the
   pan. Top with artichokes and tear over the basil, then sprinkle evenly
   with Parmesan.

5 Cook until the underside is light golden, about 2 minutes, then
   place the pan under the grill until the top is set, about 1–2 minutes,
   and serve.

FETA, OLIVE & DILL FRITTATA

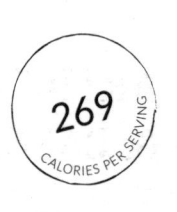

269 CALORIES PER SERVING

Gluten-free

NUTRITIONAL INFO PER SERVING: 20g fat, of which 8g saturates

0.3g carbohydrate, of which 0.3g sugars \\ 23g protein \\ 2.9g salt \\ 1g fibre

---

An awesome Greek-style combo. If reduced-fat feta isn't available, use ordinary feta and add 37 cals. In the absence of fresh dill, beat ½ tsp dried dill into the egg mixture.

PREP & COOK TIME: **7 MINUTES**
SERVINGS: **1 LARGE**

25g/1oz good-quality pitted black
  olives (ideally Kalamata) in brine
2 sprigs of fresh dill

2 eggs
sea salt and freshly ground
  black pepper
spray oil
50g/1¾oz reduced-fat feta cheese

1 | Slice or quarter the olives and pluck the dill from the main stem.

2 | In a small bowl, beat the eggs, salt and pepper with a fork until well mixed.

3 | Heat a grillproof non-stick frying pan over a medium heat and spray 4 times with spray oil. Preheat the grill to high.

4 | Pour the egg mixture into the pan and swirl to meet the edge of the pan. Scatter the olives and dill over the egg, then crumble over the feta.

5 | Cook until the underside is light golden, about 2 minutes, then place the pan under the grill until the top is set, about 1–2 minutes. Serve.

BREAKFAST BURRITO

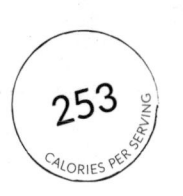

253

CALORIES PER SERVING

NUTRITIONAL INFO PER SERVING: 8g fat, of which 3g saturates
31g carbohydrate, of which 1g sugars \\ 15g protein \\ 1.2g salt \\ 4g fibre

---

This might be rather a high-calorie choice for breakfast unless you are fasting until dinnertime, but this needn't be reserved for breakfast only – it's perfect for lunch or supper and can be supplemented with salad or steamed veggies later in the day. It's the tortilla that tallies up the bulk of the calories here, so try to find one scoring around 100 cals. Tortillas store well in the freezer – grab one as you need it, and it will thaw in just a couple of minutes at room temperature.

PREP & COOK TIME: **7 MINUTES**
SERVINGS: **1 MEDIUM**

1 tortilla
20g/¾oz light cream cheese
50g/1¾oz canned fat-free refried beans
chilli powder, cayenne pepper or taco seasoning, to taste

1 egg
sea salt and freshly ground black pepper
spray oil
Mexican salsa, to serve (optional, about 20 cals for 2 tbsp)

1   Place the tortilla on a microwave-safe plate. Spread with the cream
    cheese – not too thinly, leaving some creamy lumps. Dab the refried
    beans over the cheese and spread out slightly with a fork. Sprinkle with
    chilli powder and set aside.

2   Heat a non-stick frying pan over a medium–high heat. Crack the egg
    into a small bowl and season with salt and pepper. Beat briefly with a
    fork, so that the yolk is broken but some white is still visible.

3   Spray the pan 4 times with spray oil. Pour in the egg and swirl to reach
    the edges of the pan. Once the bottom is set, fold and stir lightly until
    cooked to your liking, about 1 minute, then remove the pan from the
    heat.

4   Place the tortilla in the microwave and cook on high power for
    30–45 seconds, until just heated through – test a patch of beans with
    your fingertip (overcooking will toughen the tortilla).

5   Scoop the egg onto the tortilla and roll up. Spoon over the salsa
    (if using) and serve.

CHAPTER 7
SIMPLE SNACKS

SOME FASTERS choose never to snack on fast days because they find it makes them hungrier. Others find ultra-low-calorie snacks a godsend for a light grazing approach to fasting. Either way, as long as you count the calories in your snacks (however small), you are still succeeding at fasting as defined by the parameters of 5:2.

The ideas and recipes in this chapter can also be put together to make a meal, adding protein such as egg or tofu where necessary, or a baked potato with cottage cheese or yogurt.

Super simple snacks
- Celery sticks with Mexican salsa for dipping – celery: about 6 cals for 1 large stalk; salsa: about 27 cals per 100g – check the label and weigh out a 50–100g dipping bowl.

- Thick cucumber slices with pickled sushi ginger – 10 cals per ¼ large cucumber.

- Cucumber wedges with lime juice, salt and chilli powder or taco seasoning mix – 10 cals per ¼ large cucumber.

- Sauerkraut – about 20 cals per 100g.

- Pickles: gherkins, onions, garlic, jalapeños – about 23 cals per 100g.

- Frozen grape pops – choose large, red seedless grapes and drive cocktail sticks through them, then freeze in a bag – about 3 calories each.

- Apple wedges dipped in an ultra-low-calorie sugar substitute such as Splenda® or Truvia® mixed with cinnamon – 52 cals per 100g apple.

- Chat (or chaat) masala – this salty, tangy, hot Indian spice mix is specially designed to be sprinkled over fruit and veg. It's calorie-free and brings life to celery, cucumbers, tomatoes, apple wedges and mango chunks. It's also yummy with low-fat cottage cheese and yogurt. Use it also as a seasoning for salads, potatoes, stews, soups and bean dishes. Find it online or in Asian food shops.

MARINATED CRUDITÉS

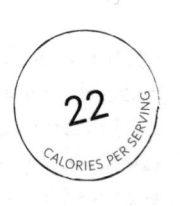

22 CALORIES PER SERVING

Gluten-free \\ Dairy-free \\ Vegan
NUTRITIONAL INFO PER SERVING: 0.3g fat, of which trace saturates
4g carbohydrate, of which 4g sugars \\ 1g protein \\ 0.9g salt \\ 2g fibre

Here's a trick for transforming a batch of crunchy marinated veggies from dull to desirable by employing salt, lemon, and a little time. It makes a substantial batch which adds up to a total of about 120 cals for over a pound of veg, so you can nibble away freely without having to count much. They will keep in the fridge for 3 days, so it's likely you can spread them over 2 fast days (and non-fast days). As well as being a low-cal stomach filler, they give you the nutrient and fibre benefits of raw veg – a real health tonic.

PREP & COOK TIME: **10 MINUTES,**
PLUS 3–4 HOURS MARINATING
SERVINGS: **ABOUT 6**

½ red pepper, cored
½ yellow pepper, cored

150g/5½oz white cabbage
100g/3½oz courgette (zucchini)
100g/3½oz celery
50g/1¾oz sugar snap peas
1 tbsp sea salt
1 tbsp fresh lemon juice

1 | Cut all the veg into strips or bite-sized chunks. Place in a bowl and sprinkle with the salt. Toss with your hands to coat evenly.

2 | Transfer to a colander and place over a bowl. Cover with clingfilm and refrigerate, stirring occasionally, for 3–4 hours.

3 | Shake the veg in the colander to drain thoroughly (do not rinse). Place the veg in a clean bowl, add the lemon juice, and stir.

4 | Cover and store in the fridge, ideally in a container with a tight-fitting lid so you can shake occasionally, using the juices to dress the veg.

\\ Keep in an airtight container in the fridge for up to 3 days. Not suitable for freezing.

COTTAGE CHEESE LETTUCE CUPS

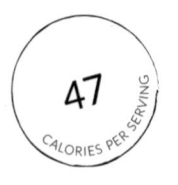

47 CALORIES PER SERVING

Gluten-free

NUTRITIONAL INFO PER SERVING: 0.9g fat, of which 0.5g saturates
3g carbohydrate, of which 3g sugars \\ 7g protein \\ 0.6g salt \\ 0.6g fibre

Deliver these straight to your mouth with your fingers.

PREP & COOK TIME: 2 MINUTES
SERVINGS: 1

2 Little Gem lettuce leaves
50g/1¾oz/¼ cup low-fat cottage
   cheese

2 pickled jalapeño slices and/or 1 sliced
   pickled onion
freshly ground black pepper

Place the lettuce leaves on a plate and divide the cottage cheese evenly between them. Top with pickled jalapeños or pickled onions and grind over some pepper.

MARINATED WATER CHESTNUTS

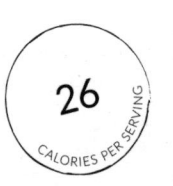

26 CALORIES PER SERVING

Gluten-free (if gluten-free soy sauce is used) \\ Dairy-free \\ Vegan

NUTRITIONAL INFO PER SERVING: 0g fat, of which 0g saturates

6g carbohydrate, of which 3g sugars \\ 0.8g protein \\ 1.4g salt \\ 2g fibre

---

Three ingredients that add up to more than the sum of their parts. Crunchy and hugely flavourful – and you can munch away almost calorie-freely.

PREP & COOK TIME: **5 MINUTES**
PLUS 2 HOURS OR OVERNIGHT CHILLING
SERVINGS: **2 LARGE**

140g/5oz canned water chestnuts
  (1 x 225g can, drained)
1 tbsp dark soy sauce
1 tsp seasoned rice vinegar or
  sushi vinegar

1. Simply combine everything in a bowl or a zip-seal bag and mix well.

2. Refrigerate for an hour or two, or overnight.

\\ These can also be added to a salad, a bowl of noodles, or a stir-fry.

\\ Keep in an airtight container in the fridge for up to 3 days. Not suitable for freezing.

CURRIED COTTAGE CHEESE

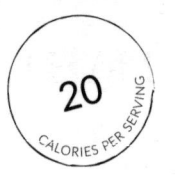

20 CALORIES PER SERVING

Gluten-free

NUTRITIONAL INFO PER SERVING: (2 tbsp serving) 0.4g fat, of which 0.2g saturates 0.8g carbohydrate, of which 0.8g sugars \\ 3g protein \\ 0.2g salt \\ 0g fibre

Spoon this into Little Gem lettuce cups or scoop it up with celery sticks.

PREP & COOK TIME: **2 MINUTES**
SERVINGS: **2**

50g/1¾oz/¼ cup low-fat cottage cheese

1 tsp fresh lemon juice
¼ tsp curry powder
sea salt
cayenne pepper, to taste

Stir everything together in a small bowl. Taste for seasoning and enjoy with raw veggies.

\\ Keep in an airtight container in the fridge for up to 3 days.

LIGHT RANCH DIP

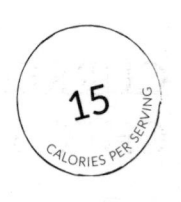

15
CALORIES PER SERVING

Gluten-free

NUTRITIONAL INFO PER SERVING: (2 tbsp serving) 0.2g fat, of which 0.2g saturates
2g carbohydrate, of which 2g sugars \\ 1g protein \\ trace salt \\ 0g fibre

---

Here's a speedy concoction to give extra flavour to celery sticks or any prepared raw veggie. It also tastes good with pickled gherkins dipped in, and can be used as a salad dressing.

PREP & COOK TIME: **3 MINUTES**
SERVINGS: **2**

50g/1¾oz/3 tbsp low-fat yogurt
1 tsp white wine vinegar

¼ tsp garlic powder or granules
¼ tsp dried dill
sea salt and freshly ground
   black pepper

Stir everything together in a small bowl. Taste for seasoning and enjoy with raw veggies.

\\ Keep in an airtight container in the fridge for up to 3 days.

SPICED PICKLED ONIONS

CALORIES PER SERVING (4 ONIONS) 14

Gluten-free \\ Dairy-free \\ Vegan

NUTRITIONAL INFO PER SERVING: 0.1g fat, of which trace saturates

3g carbohydrate, of which 2g sugars \\ 0.6g protein \\ 0.7g salt \\ 1g fibre

Here's one of my tricks for turning a jar of store-bought economy pickled onions into something addictive. Look for a large jar without added sugar or oil, at around 40 cals per 100g. The whole spices below are only suggestions – raid your spice cupboard, or buy a mix of whole pickling spices. After about a week of spicy mingling, the onions will taste exotic and irresistible.

PREP & COOK TIME: **5 MINUTES, PLUS 1 WEEK MARINATING**

SERVINGS: **ABOUT 7**

2–3 small dried chillies
1 tsp coriander seeds

1 tsp cumin seeds
2 star anise
5 whole cloves
5 cardamom pods
1 large jar (about 440g) pickled onions

1. You'll get the best flavour out of these spices by lightly toasting them, either in a dry pan over a low–medium heat, or, perhaps surprisingly, in the microwave. Put the whole spices on a microwave-safe plate and cook on high for about 15–20 seconds, or until fragrant. You may hear a bit of popping which is fine, but do be careful not to burn them.

2. Leave the spices to cool and then add to the pickled onion jar (or just add the spices without toasting them). You may have to eat a couple of onions to fit the spices in there. Replace the lid tightly and shake the jar to distribute the spices. Store in the fridge and shake daily.

3. They'll be ready in about a week, and keep indefinitely in the fridge.

FROZEN VIRGIN MARY POPS

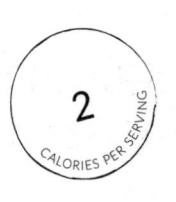

2
CALORIES PER SERVING

Gluten-free (if gluten-free soy sauce is used) \\ Dairy-free \\ Vegan
NUTRITIONAL INFO PER SERVING: 0g fat, of which 0g saturates
0.4g carbohydrate, of which 0.4g sugars \\ 0.1g protein \\ 0.1g salt \\ 0.1g fibre

Spicy little savoury frozen treats to take your mind off your next meal. Because of the salt in the recipe, these melt more quickly than frozen fruit, so have a small plate at the ready when eating.

PREP & COOK TIME: **5 MINUTES**
SERVINGS: **12**

6 cherry tomatoes, halved
150ml/5fl oz/⅔ cup tomato juice or
   vegetable juice

Optional seasonings
dark soy sauce
hot pepper sauce, such as Tabasco
fresh lemon or lime juice
chilli powder
crushed coriander seeds
freshly ground black pepper

1 Place a tomato half cut-side down in each of 12 ice-cube moulds.

2 Measure the tomato or vegetable juice into a jug. Spice up the juice to your taste with the suggested seasonings.

3 Pour the juice over the tomatoes to fill the moulds. Cover the tray tightly with clingfilm. Punch one cocktail stick per mould through the clingfilm into the tomato.

4 Freeze overnight. You may need a knife to dislodge the frozen pop.

\\ Keep frozen and use within 3 months.

FROZEN PEACH & RASPBERRY POPS

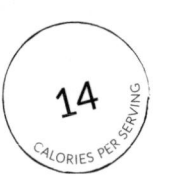

14 CALORIES PER SERVING

Gluten-free \\ Dairy-free \\ Vegan
NUTRITIONAL INFO PER SERVING: 0g fat, of which 1g saturates
0g carbohydrate, of which 3g sugars \\ 0.3g protein \\ 0g salt \\ 0.5g fibre

---

Frozen fruity fun for idle mouths!

PREP & COOK TIME: **5 MINUTES**
SERVINGS: **12**

1 x 400g can sliced peaches in
natural juice
12 raspberries

1   Tip the peaches into a sieve over a measuring jug and reserve the juice.

2   Place one raspberry each, open-end down, in 12 ice-cube moulds.

3   Place a peach slice over the top of the raspberry, then top up each mould with juice.

4   Cover the tray tightly with clingfilm. Punch one cocktail stick per mould through the clingfilm into the fruit.

5   Freeze overnight. You may need a knife to help dislodge the frozen pop.

\\ Keep frozen and use within 3 months.

CHAPTER 8
DRINKS & APPETITE CRUSHERS

THIS MAY SOUND patently obvious, but don't forget that everything you drink has to be counted in your fast-day allowance – that includes lattes, fruit juice and alcohol. So give those high-cal options a miss two days a week and fill up on water-based hydration.

The importance of staying hydrated on fast days can't be emphasized enough. We get a surprisingly large amount of water from our food, so by cutting that back, we're also cutting back on hydration. Drinking water also helps you stay full and staves off hunger pangs. Two litres a day is the bare minimum, but aim for more.

Admittedly, tap water can be pretty boring. Chilling it in bottles or a large lidded fridge jug makes it a bit more enjoyable. A drink with some flavour can be much more satisfying for idle taste buds, especially when you are feeling hungry, but it's best to keep it calorie-free, or close to it.

Hot tea and coffee can be sipped throughout the day on fast days – but remember, no milk or sugar. Sometimes I feel I just can't live without my usual morning cuppa with semi-skimmed milk and agave nectar, but at about 50 calories, that's a whopping 10% of my daily allowance, so I usually try to abstain. Sometimes it is worth it, but I always log it in to my fast-day diary. A low-calorie hot chocolate drink (around 40 cals) can be a soothing bedtime drink and lots of fasters look forward to it as a soporific treat. Valerian tea, lemon verbena and other herbal sleep-inducing mixtures – with a spoonful of honey (around 21 cals per tsp) if you can afford the calories – can also help.

There are a whole host of teas that have been reported to help with weight loss, either by increasing metabolism, flushing out impurities with diuretic properties, or suppressing appetite. Green tea is one of them, and this is a favourite hot tea for me on fast days, brewed in a 1-litre/1¾-pint teapot, with water just off the boil to preserve the antioxidants in the tea. I use 1 heaped tbsp of loose leaves, and I always add a couple of peppermint teabags or fresh mint sprigs to soften its flavour. Green tea is great for keeping you going during the day as it is high in caffeine and really sharpens the mind, but don't drink it close to bedtime.

Other teas that are reported to benefit weight loss are liquorice (my usual choice for fridge tea), hibiscus, ginger and cinnamon.

In this chapter, you'll find suggestions for hot and cold drinks, along with some tonics that studies have shown might actively suppress appetite.

FRIDGE TEA

Since I started making this on fast days, it's become an everyday drink. I use a cleaned 2-litre/3½-pint plastic juice bottle with a wide mouth (4cm/1½in; the wide mouth makes it easy to deposit and remove the tea bags). Every evening, I fill it with fresh cold tap water and pop in 3 herbal teabags, close it tightly, shake it and leave it in the fridge overnight. In the morning, I have a delicious supply of iced herbal tea to get me through the day (I leave the bags in until refilling). I commit to drinking the whole thing, plus other liquids such as hot tea. I also use a 2-litre jug for plain water or flavoured water (see below). Any tea can be made this way – black or green too – you may wish to flavour it further with lemon juice and/or an ultra-low-calorie sugar substitute (see page 36).

FLAVOURED WATER

Here's another simple way to make water more interesting. The evening before a fast day (or in the morning), fill a 2-litre/3½-pint jug with fresh water and add slices of cucumber and sprigs of fresh mint. Try also slices of orange, lemon, lime, melon, berries, or fresh pomegranate seeds, or any combination of these. Steep in the fridge overnight and commit to drinking the lot during the day. Strain off the flavourings and funnel the flavoured water into a large water bottle if you need to take it with you.

SAVOURY DRINKS

These can be helpful not so much for hydration but for tricking your palate into thinking it's eating. Try a mug of hot vegetable stock, or yeast extract such as Marmite dissolved in boiling water. Tomato or vegetable juices are good hunger-curbers, especially if spiced up with soy sauce, lemon juice and chilli, and fairly low calorie at about 24 cals per 100ml. My favourite fast-day juice is a glass of well-chilled Turkish *şalgam suyu*, made from fermented carrots and turnips. It's a bit like drinking the juice from a pickle jar – intensely sour and salty, with a stimulating chilli burn. It's an enjoyable slap in the face that temporarily sweeps hunger aside. Plus its shocking pink colour is a thrill for the eyeballs – it's sensational all round! What's more, it's super-healthy (offering the benefits of lactic fermentation) and contains just 2 cals per 100ml. Seek it out in Turkish or Mediterranean groceries.

Other appetite crushers

- Apple cider vinegar – dilute 1 tbsp with a little water and knock it back first thing in the morning.

- Apples – renowned for curbing appetite at 52 cals per 100g.

- Hot mustard and wasabi – a small dab distracts the palate.

- Chewing gum – give your mouth something to do!

GRAPEFRUIT CRUSH

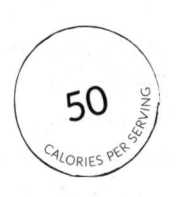

50
CALORIES PER SERVING

Gluten-free \\ Dairy-free \\ Vegan
NUTRITIONAL INFO PER SERVING: 0.2g fat, of which trace saturates
11g carbohydrate, of which 11g sugars \\ 1g protein \\ trace salt \\ 3g fibre

This rather brutal yet simple treatment of grapefruit eliminates the tedious task of pre-loosening each section with a knife. Studies have shown that grapefruit is a weight-loss aid, curbing appetite and possibly lowering insulin levels. I've found that this keeps hunger at bay for a good few hours.

PREP & COOK TIME: **3 MINUTES**
SERVINGS: **1 LARGE**

1 medium grapefruit (about 160g/5½oz), chilled

1   Slice the grapefruit in half equatorially. Flick out any visible seeds with a fork. Hold half cut-side down over a jug or a bowl and squeeze the living daylights out of it, then use the fork to scrape out all the soft, juicy flesh you can. Repeat with the second half.

2   Most remaining seeds will float to the top, so fish them out. Pour into a glass or your favourite teacup. Sip and scoop the flesh mouthward with a small spoon.

CHIA SEED JELLY TONIC

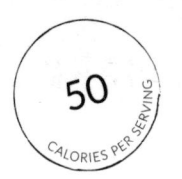

50
CALORIES PER SERVING

Gluten-free \\ Dairy-free \\ Vegan

NUTRITIONAL INFO PER SERVING: 3g fat, of which 0.3g saturates

4g carbohydrate, of which 0g sugars \\ 2g protein \\ 0g salt \\ 3g fibre

---

Chia seeds (available from health food retailers) are gaining popularity in the superfood stakes; they are allegedly endowed with powers to suppress appetite, benefit heart health and reduce inflammation, and provide high levels of complete protein, omega oils, and a host of vitamins and minerals. The seed originates in Mexico, and chia is an Aztec word meaning strength – allegedly the Aztecs consumed chia to fuel long journeys on foot and before going into battle. Since they absorb nine times their volume in liquid, it follows that soaking them long enough to make them edible will curb hunger, as they continue to swell in your stomach, while delivering their nutritional benefits.

I won't pretend this tonic is delicious. The seeds turn the liquid slightly jelly-like and look weird – just knock it back quickly, you know it will do you good! Adding a bit of no-sugar-added squash to the water will make it more appetizing. You could also soak the seeds in milk, soy milk, or juice – just be sure to count the extra calories.

PREP & COOK TIME: 1 MINUTE,
PLUS 15 MINUTES STANDING
SERVINGS: 1

2 tsp chia seeds
100ml/3½fl oz/scant ½ cup water

1 | Place the chia seeds in a screwtop jar and top up with liquid. Close the jar and shake vigorously.

2 | Leave to soak for 15 minutes, shaking once or twice. Shake again, then gulp it down, chewing slightly as you go.

FIERY TEA TONIC

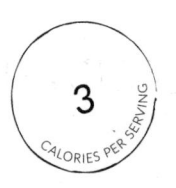

3

CALORIES PER SERVING

Gluten-free \\ Dairy-free \\ Vegan
NUTRITIONAL INFO PER SERVING: 0g fat, of which 0g saturates
0.4g carbohydrate, of which 0.2g sugars \\ 0.1g protein \\ 0g salt \\ 0g fibre

This calorie-free version of hot honey and lemon has a chilli kick, which boosts your metabolism and is reputed to keep hunger at bay. It's also a great remedy for a head cold.

PREP & COOK TIME: **2 MINUTES**
SERVINGS: **1**

⅛ tsp cayenne pepper
1 tbsp fresh lemon or lime juice
ultra-low-calorie sugar substitute,
   to taste

1 Boil the kettle.

2 Place the cayenne pepper and lemon or lime juice in your favourite mug and top up with boiling water.

3 Add sweetener to taste and stir well.

ICED ALMOND
TEA COOLER

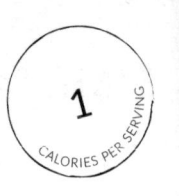

1

CALORIES PER SERVING

Gluten-free \\ Dairy-free \\ Vegan

NUTRITIONAL INFO PER SERVING: 0g fat, of which 0g saturates

0.2g carbohydrate, of which 0.2g sugars \\ 0g protein \\ 0g salt \\ 0g fibre

---

Fridge-steeped iced tea is an easy fast-day drink – use 2 teabags per litre of water and chill overnight, then add lemon and sweetener to taste, and pour over ice. Here's a jazzed-up version with almond and vanilla essences. Depending on what type of almond extract you use, the cooler may have a slightly oily appearance, which is from the natural almond oil.

PREP & COOK TIME: **2 MINUTES,**
PLUS OVERNIGHT STEEPING
SERVINGS: **4**

1 litre/1¾ pints/4 cups cold water
2 teabags (ordinary black tea)

3 tbsp fresh lemon or lime juice
¼ tsp pure almond extract
¼ tsp pure vanilla extract
ultra-low-calorie sugar substitute,
  to taste
ice

1. Place the cold water in a lidded container suitable for pouring. Add the teabags, close the lid and shake, then refrigerate overnight.

2. Remove the teabags.

3. Add lemon juice, almond and vanilla extracts, and sweetener to taste. Pour over ice.

LIME & MINT SLUSH

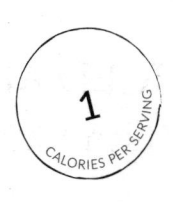

1 CALORIES PER SERVING

Gluten-free \\ Dairy-free \\ Vegan
NUTRITIONAL INFO PER SERVING: 0g fat, of which 0g saturates
0.4g carbohydrate, of which 0.4g sugars \\ 0g protein \\ 0g salt \\ 0g fibre

---

This cooling, summery slush will stay partially frozen in the fridge for a good few hours, and is also refreshing once melted. The calories are negligible, so sip away to your heart's content.

PREP & COOK TIME: **3 MINUTES**
SERVINGS: **4**

ice
leaves stripped from 3 fresh
  mint sprigs
2 tbsp fresh lime juice
3 tbsp ultra-low-calorie sugar
  substitute, or to taste

1   Fill your blender half full with ice. Top up with cold water to two-thirds full.

2   Add the mint, lime juice and sweetener.

3   Whizz at high speed until slushy. Taste and whizz in more lime or sweetener if desired.

CHAPTER 9
CONVENIENCE FOODS
& PACKED LUNCHES

FOR SOME FAST-DAY MEALS, you may not want to cook or are unable to because you're at work or elsewhere. That's when ready-made food and packed lunches come in, but don't forget to calculate the calories and log them in your fast-day diary.

Fortunately, convenience foods usually have the calories stated on the label. If they don't, it's a bit risky to guess, so on fast days, be sure to eat or buy labelled food – forget about eating at a restaurant unless you can count the calories accurately. You'll be amazed how many calories the average supermarket sandwich contains, but you needn't waste your whole day's calorie allowance on just one sandwich.

MY TOP SOUP TRICK

Soup, out of a can or a carton, can easily be jazzed up to make it seem a bit more like homemade. This works particularly well with low-calorie lentil or bean-based soups, which tend to be more filling and higher in protein than vegetable-based soups. My personal favourite is a supermarket own-label 'Moroccan chickpea' soup, which comes in a standard 400g can at 134 calories for the lot. I empty the whole can into a saucepan and heat just to simmering. I grab a big handful of baby spinach (about 50g – 12 calories) and stir it into the soup. Using scissors, I snip the spinach in the soup as it wilts to chop it up. Once it's wilted, I transfer the soup to a bowl, splodge a large dollop of low-fat yogurt on top (27 cals), dribble over some chilli sauce, and sprinkle with ras-el-hanout, then finally add a squeeze of lemon juice. *Voilà*, a massive, delicious, healthy meal for just 173 cals!

OTHER GOOD FAST-DAY CONVENIENCE FOODS

- Canned ratatouille – a 400g can has around 140 cals and at least 2 of your 5-a-day veg.

- Canned French onion soup (check the label to be sure it's vegetarian) makes a rich and satisfying base – just add steamed veggies.

- Reduced-calorie baked beans – spice up with curry powder, garam masala or ras-el-hanout.

- Vegetarian chilli.

- Instant soup packets – on fast days, sometimes they just hit the spot and are usually around 80 cals or fewer.

- Soy-based vegetarian hot dogs – eat with heaps of sauerkraut and a smear of hot mustard.

- Soy-based veggie burgers – with salad, no bun.

FAST-DAY LUNCH BOXES

The following recipes are perfectly portable.

TO EAT COLD:

Black-Eyed Pea & Coconut Salad (page 52)
Broad Bean & Basil Puree Platter (page 43)
Cold Cucumber Soup with Walnuts (page 59)
Courgette & Feta Frittata (page 78)
Creamy Potato & Egg Salad (keep dressing separate) (page 46)
Greek-style Butterbeans with Herbs & Tomatoes (page 88)
Mango & Black Bean Salad (page 51)
Micro-Broccoli Salad with Sweet Seed Clusters & Egg (page 54)
Miso Aubergine & Tofu with Red Cabbage Salad (page 55)
Neon Red Pepper Soup (page 66)
Raw Cauliflower & Feta Tabbouleh (page 44)
Spiced Gazpacho with Lemony Egg (keep egg separate) (page 57)
Spicy Palm Heart & Egg Salad (keep dressing separate) (page 47)
Sweet & Sour Tofu & Pineapple (page 97)
Thai Salad Wraps with Chargrilled Tofu (leave out the lettuce cups and combine the rest of the salad) (page 49)

TO REHEAT:

Butterbean & Rosemary Soup (page 64)
Greek-style Butterbeans with Herbs & Tomatoes (page 88)
Green Gumbo with Parmesan (page 94)
Minted Chickpea Soup (page 61)
Miraculously Rich Hotpot (page 100)
Neon Red Pepper Soup (page 66)
Pappa al Pomodoro (keep bread separate) (page 68)
Saffron Celeriac & Puy Lentil Bowl (page 102)
South Indian Egg & Coconut Curry (page 108)
South Indian Mango Curry (page 106)
South Indian Tofu & Mushroom Curry (page 110)
Spicy Egyptian Bean Soup (page 65)

Sweet & Sour Bean & Beetroot Stew (page 92)
Sweet & Sour Tofu & Pineapple (page 97)
Sweet Lentil Cabbage Wraps (page 82)
Vegetable & Chick Pea Tagine (page 90)

OTHER LUNCHBOX IDEAS

- Make Light Ranch Dip (page 191), Egg & Parmesan Dressing (page 149), or Creamy Sesame Sauce (page 156). Pack raw crudités and Little Gem lettuce hearts for dipping, plus a hard-boiled egg and 2 wholegrain melba toast crackers with a wedge of low-fat spreadable cheese, plus a few grapes.

- Bring the components for a Caesar-esque salad: Egg & Parmesan Dressing (page 149), hearts of romaine or Little Gem lettuce, a hard-boiled egg, wholegrain melba toasts to crush as croutons, and a little extra Parmesan if desired.

- Make a cucumber sandwich using low-cal wholemeal bread spread sparingly with light cream cheese – sprinkle with a pinch of dried dill, salt and pepper; supplement with celery sticks and Mexican salsa for dipping and a couple of pickled gherkins.

- See Chapter 7, Simple Snacks, for further ideas to use as the building blocks of a packed lunch.

INDEX   GF = gluten-free   DF = dairy-free

almond(s)
  banana almond smoothie (GF) 165
  cinnamon almond porridge (DF) 163
  iced almond tea cooler (GF/DF) 204
  & tomato sauce (GF/DF) 155–6
appetite crushers 200
apple cinnamon porridge (DF) 161–2
artichoke hearts 28
artichokes
  artichoke, Parmesan & basil frittata (GF) 180
  caramelized (GF/DF) 138–9
Asian dressing (GF) 150–1
aubergines
  miso aubergine & tofu with red cabbage salad (GF/DF) 55–6

baked jacket potatoes *see* jacket potatoes
banana almond smoothie (GF) 165
basil
  artichoke, Parmesan & basil frittata (GF) 180
  broad bean & basil puree platter (GF) 43–4
BBQ marinade for tofu (GF/DF) 142–3
beans 28
  black-eyed pea & coconut salad (GF/DF) 52–3
  breakfast burrito 182–3
  broad bean & basil puree platter (GF) 43–4
  butterbean & rosemary soup (GF/DF) 64–5
  Georgian-style beans in walnut & coriander sauce (GF/DF) 86–7
  Greek-style butterbeans with herbs & tomatoes (GF/DF) 88–9
  mango & black bean salad (GF/DF) 51–2
  spicy Egyptian bean soup (GF/DF) 65–6
  spicy Mexican bean flatbread 76
  sweet & sour bean & beetroot stew (GF/DF) 92–3
beetroot
  sweet & sour bean & beetroot stew (GF/DF) 92–3
black beans
  mango & black bean salad (GF/DF) 51–2
black-eyed pea & coconut salad (GF/DF) 52–3
bread
  dill & garlic tomatoes on cheese toast 170
  eggs in a frame 171
  see also flatbread
breakfast burrito 182–3
breakfast miso cup (GF/DF) 168
broad bean & basil puree platter (GF) 43–4
broccoli
  micro-broccoli salad with sweet seed clusters & egg (GF/DF) 54–5
  teriyaki tofu & roasted (GF/DF) 99–100
butterbean(s)
  Greek-style butterbeans with herbs & tomatoes (GF/DF) 88–9
  & rosemary soup (GF/DF) 64–5

cabbage
  miso aubergine & tofu with red cabbage salad (GF/DF) 55–6
  Spanish stir-fry with cumin-yogurt sauce (GF) 72–3

sweet lentil cabbage wraps (GF/LF) 82–3
capers 37
  puttanesca sauce (GF/DF) 153–4
  roasted tempeh with crisp (GF/DF) 144–5
  spicy Mexican bean flatbread 76
caramelized artichokes (GF/DF) 138–9
carrot juice
  hotpot (GF/DF) 100–1
casserole, sweet potato & palm heart (GF/
  DF) 104–5
cauliflower
  chargrilled cauliflower slab (GF/DF)
    119–20
  couscous (GF/DF) 118–19
  Greek-style egg & lemon soup with saffron
    (GF/DF) 62–3
  Parmesan pancakes (GF) 120–1
  raw cauliflower & feta tabbouleh (GF/DF)
    44–5
cayenne pepper 35
celeriac
  saffron celeriac and puy lentil bowl (GF/
    DF) 102–3
celery 186
chargrilled cauliflower slab (GF/DF) 119–20
chat masala 186
cheese 33
  artichoke, Parmesan & basil frittata (GF)
    180
  cauliflower Parmesan pancakes (GF)
    120–1
  courgette & feta frittata (GF) 78–9
  creamy chilli & sweetcorn frittata (GF)
    178–9
  dill & garlic tomatoes on cheese toast 170

egg & Parmesan dressing (GF) 149–50
  feta, olive & dill frittata (GF) 181
  green gumbo with Parmesan (DF) 94–5
  & herb scramble (GF) 175
  raw cauliflower & feta tabbouleh (GF/DF)
    44–5
  three-tomato & mozzarella flatbread 74–5
  see also cottage cheese; cream cheese
cheesy courgette & dill pancakes 77–8
chia seed jelly tonic (GF/DF) 202
chickpeas
  minted chickpea soup (GF/DF) 61
  Spanish stir-fry with cumin-yogurt sauce
    (GF) 72–3
  vegetable & chickpea tagine (GF/DF) 90–1
chillies 35
  creamy chilli sweetcorn frittata (GF)
    178–9
  hot & sour tofu bowl (GF/DF) 96–7
  Mexican scramble (GF) 176
chocolate velvet smoothie (GF) 164
cinnamon
  almond porridge (DF) 162
  apple cinnamon porridge (DF) 161–2
coconut
  black-eyed pea & coconut salad (GF/DF)
    52–3
  South Indian egg & coconut curry (GF)
    108–9
coffee
  iced mocha frappé (GF) 167
cold cucumber soup with walnuts (GF)
  59–60
convenience foods 208–9

coriander
  Georgian-style beans in walnut &
    coriander sauce (GF/DF) 86–7
  green lightning salsa (GF/DF) 146–7
cottage cheese
  cheesy courgette & dill pancakes 77–8
  curried (GF) 190
  lettuce cups (GF) 188
courgette(s)
  cheesy courgette & dill pancakes 77–8
  & feta frittata (GF) 78–9
  Greek-style egg & lemon soup with saffron
    (GF/DF) 62–3
couscous, cauliflower (GF/DF) 118–19
cream cheese
  breakfast burrito 182–3
  creamy mushroom caps (GF) 169
creamy chilli sweetcorn frittata (GF) 178–9
creamy mushroom caps (GF) 169
creamy paprika mushrooms (GF) 80–1
creamy potato & egg salad (GF) 46–7
creamy sesame sauce (GF) 156–7
creamy spiked spinach (GF) 136–7
crudités, marinated (GF/DF) 187–8
crushed potatoes (GF/DF) 125
cucumbers 186
  cold cucumber soup with walnuts (GF)
    59–60
cumin
  black-eyed pea & coconut salad (GF/DF)
    52–3
  Spanish stir-fry with cumin-yogurt sauce
    (GF) 72–3
  spiced gazpacho with lemony egg (GF/
    DF) 57–8
  spicy palm heart & egg salad (GF/DF) 47–8
  -yogurt dressing 51–2

curried cottage cheese (GF) 190
curries
  South Indian egg & coconut (GF) 108–9
  South Indian mango (GF) 106–7
  South Indian tofu & mushroom (GF/DF)
    110–11

dill
  cheesy courgette & dill pancakes 77–8
  feta, olive & dill frittata (GF) 181
  & garlic tomatoes on cheese toast 170
dips
  broad bean & basil puree platter (GF)
    43–4
  light ranch (GF) 191
dressings
  cumin-yogurt 51–2
  egg & Parmesan (GF) 149–50
  magic Asian (GF/DF) 150–1
dried mushrooms 36
drinks
  chia seed jelly tonic (GF/DF) 202
  fiery tea tonic (GF/DF) 203
  flavoured water 199
  fridge tea 199
  grapefruit crush (GF/DF) 201
  iced almond tea cooler (GF/DF) 204
  lime & mint slush (GF/DF) 205
  savoury 200
  see also frappés; smoothies

egg(s) 33
  breakfast burrito 182–3
  creamy potato & egg salad (GF) 46–7
  in a frame 171
  Greek-style egg & lemon soup with saffron
    (GF/DF) 62–3

micro-broccoli salad with sweet seed
  clusters & (GF/DF) 54–5
& Parmesan dressing (GF) 149–50
poached (GF/DF) 133
poached in red pepper sauce (GF/DF)
  84–5
South Indian egg & coconut curry (GF)
  108–9
spiced gazpacho with lemony (GF/DF)
  57–8
spicy palm heart & egg salad (GF/DF) 47–8
  strand noodles (GF/DF) 131–2
see also frittatas; omelettes;
  scrambled eggs

feta cheese
  courgette & feta frittata (GF) 78–9
  feta, olive & dill frittata (GF) 181
  raw cauliflower & feta tabbouleh (GF/DF)
    44–5
fiery tea tonic (GF/DF) 203
flatbread 74
  spicy Mexican bean 76
  three-tomato & mozzarella 74–5
flavoured water 199
frappés
  iced mocha (GF) 167
  mango and ginger frappé (GF) 166
fridge tea 199
frittatas 178
  artichoke, Parmesan & basil (GF) 180
  courgette & feta (GF) 78–9
  creamy chilli sweetcorn (GF) 178–9
  feta, olive & dill (GF) 181
frozen grape pops 186
frozen peach & raspberry pops (GF/DF) 194
frozen veg 29

frozen Virgin Mary pops (GF/DF) 193
fruit 29

garlic 36
  dill & garlic tomatoes on cheese toast 170
  mushrooms (GF/DF) 135–6
gazpacho
  spiced gazpacho with lemony egg (GF/
    DF) 57–8
Georgian-style beans in walnut & coriander
  sauce (GF/DF) 86–7
ginger 36
  mango and ginger frappé (GF) 166
grapefruit crush (GF/DF) 201
grapes
  frozen grape pops 186
Greek-style butterbeans with herbs &
  tomatoes (GF/DF) 88–9
Greek-style egg & lemon soup with saffron
  (GF/DF) 62–3
green gumbo with Parmesan (DF) 94–5
green lightning salsa (GF/DF) 146
gumbo
  green gumbo with Parmesan (DF) 94–5

herbs 36
  cheese & herb scramble (GF) 175
  Greek-style butterbeans with herbs &
    tomatoes (GF/DF) 88–9
hot and sour tofu bowl (GF/DF) 96–7
hotpot (GF/DF) 100–1

iced almond tea cooler (GF/DF) 204
iced mocha frappé (GF) 167
Indian omelette roll (GF/DF) 129–30

jacket potatoes 122
  microwave-baked (GF/DF) 124
  oven-baked (GF/DF) 122–3

kidney beans
  Georgian-style beans in walnut &
    coriander sauce (GF/DF) 86–7
  sweet & sour bean & beetroot stew (GF/
    DF) 92–3
kohlrabi
  Thai salad wraps with chargrilled tofu (GF/
    DF) 49–50

leeks
  Greek-style egg & lemon soup with saffron
    (GF/DF) 62–3
lemons 33
  fiery tea tonic (GF/DF) 203
  Greek-style egg & lemon soup with saffron
    (GF/DF) 62–3
  spiced gazpacho with lemony egg (GF/
    DF) 57–8
lentils 28
  saffron celeriac and puy lentil bowl (GF/
    DF) 102–3
  sweet lentil cabbage wraps (GF/DF) 82–3
lettuce
  cottage cheese lettuce cups (GF) 188
light ranch dip (GF) 191
lime(s) 33
  & mint slush (GF/DF) 205

magic Asian dressing (GF/DF) 150–1
mango(es)
  & black bean salad (GF/DF) 51–2
  and ginger frappé (GF) 166
  South Indian mango curry (GF) 106–7

marinades
  piquant marinade for tofu (GF/DF) 140–1
  smoky BBQ marinade for tofu (GF/DF)
    142–3
marinated crudités (GF/DF) 187–8
marinated water chestnuts (GF/DF) 189
meaty tofu mini-fillets (GF/DF) 139–40
Mexican scramble (GF) 176
micro-broccoli salad with sweet seed
    clusters & egg (GF/DF) 54–5
minted chickpea soup (GF/DF) 61
miso 32
  aubergine & tofu with red cabbage salad
    (GF/DF) 55–6
  breakfast miso cup (GF/DF) 168
  noodle bowl (GF/DF) 69–70
mozzarella
  three-tomato & mozzarella flatbread 74–5
mushrooms 36
  creamy mushroom caps (GF) 169
  creamy paprika (GF) 80–1
  garlic (GF/DF) 135–6
  hotpot (GF/DF) 100–1
  South Indian tofu & mushroom curry (GF/
    DF) 110–11
  Spanish stir-fry with cumin-yogurt sauce
    (GF) 72–3
mustard 37

Napoli sauce (GF/DF) 151–2
neon red pepper soup (GF/DF) 66–7
noodles 34
  egg strand (GF/DF) 131–2
  miso noodle bowl (GF/DF) 69–70
  shirataki 116–17
nuts 37
  almond & tomato sauce (GF/DF) 155–6

cold cucumber soup with walnuts (GF) 59–60

Georgian-style beans in walnut & coriander sauce (GF/DF) 86–7

green lightning salsa (GF/DF) 146–7

oils 34

olives 37

feta, olive & dill frittata (GF) 181

puttanesca sauce (GF/DF) 153–4

omelettes

Indian omelette roll (GF/DF) 129–30

one-egg (GF/DF) 126–7

sesame omelette roll (GF/DF) 128–9

see also frittatas

onion(s)

ceviche (GF/DF) 147–8

spiced pickled onions (GF/DF) 192

palm heart(s) 28

scramble (GF/DF) 177

spicy palm heart & egg salad (GF/DF) 47–8

sweet potato & palm heart casserole (GF/DF) 104–5

pancakes

cauliflower Parmesan (GF) 120–1

cheesy courgette & dill 77–8

pappa al pomodoro (DF) 68–9

paprika

creamy paprika mushrooms (GF) 80–1

Parmesan 33

artichoke, Parmesan & basil frittata (GF) 180

cauliflower Parmesan pancakes (GF) 120–1

egg & Parmesan dressing (GF) 149–50

green gumbo with (DF) 94–5

peaches

frozen peach & raspberry pops (GF/DF) 194

peppers

eggs poached in red pepper sauce (GF/DF) 84–5

neon red pepper soup (GF/DF) 66–7

pickled onions, spiced (GF/DF) 192

pickles 29

pineapple

sweet and sour tofu & (GF/DF) 97–8

piquant marinade for tofu (GF/DF) 140–1

poached eggs (GF/DF) 133

porridge 161

apple cinnamon (DF) 161–2

cinnamon almond (DF) 162

strawberry vanilla (DF) 163

potatoes 122

creamy potato & egg salad (GF) 46–7

crushed (GF/DF) 125

jacket see jacket potatoes

sweet potato & palm heart casserole (GF/DF) 104

protein powder 37

puttanesca sauce (GF/DF) 153–4

puy lentils

saffron celeriac and puy lentil bowl (GF/DF) 102–3

raspberries

peach & raspberry pops (GF/DF) 194

raw cauliflower & feta tabbouleh (GF/DF) 44–5

red cabbage

miso aubergine & tofu with red cabbage salad (GF/DF) 55–6

red peppers see peppers

refried beans 28
  breakfast burrito 182–3
  spicy Mexican bean flatbread 76
roasted tempeh with crisp capers (GF/DF)
  144–5
rosemary
  butterbean & rosemary soup (GF/DF)
  64–5

saffron
  celeriac and puy lentil bowl (GF/DF)
  102–3
  Greek-style egg & lemon soup with (GF/
  DF) 62–3
salads
  black-eyed pea & coconut (GF/DF) 52–3
  creamy potato & egg (GF) 46–7
  mango & black bean (GF/DF) 51–2
  micro-broccoli salad with sweet seed
  clusters & egg (GF/DF) 54–5
  miso aubergine & tofu with red cabbage
  (GF/DF) 55–6
  spicy palm heart & egg (GF/DF) 47–8
  Thai salad wraps with chargrilled tofu (GF/
  DF) 49–50
salsa 37
  green lightning (GF/DF) 146–7
salt 34
sauces
  almond & tomato (GF/DF) 155–6
  creamy sesame (GF) 156–7
  cumin-yogurt 72–3
  Napoli (GF/DF) 151–2
  puttanesca (GF/DF) 153–4
sauerkraut 29, 186
  hot and sour tofu bowl (GF/DF) 96–7

savoury drinks 200
scrambled eggs 172
  cheese & herb scramble (GF) 175
  creamy (GF) 174
  fluffy (GF) 173
  Mexican scramble (GF) 176
  palm heart scramble (GF/DF) 177
sesame seeds 37
  creamy sesame sauce (GF) 156–7
  sesame omelette roll (GF/DF) 128–9
shirataki noodles 34, 116–17
smoky BBQ marinade for tofu (GF/DF)
  142–3
smoothies 164
  banana almond (GF) 165
  chocolate velvet (GF) 164
snacks, super simple 186
soups 208
  breakfast miso cup (GF/DF) 168
  butterbean & rosemary (GF/DF) 64–5
  cold cucumber soup with walnuts (GF)
  59–60
  Greek-style egg & lemon soup with saffron
  (GF/DF) 62–3
  hot and sour tofu bowl (GF/DF) 96–7
  minted chickpea (GF/DF) 61
  neon red pepper (GF/DF) 66–7
  pappa al pomodoro (DF) 68–9
  spiced gazpacho with lemony egg (GF/
  DF) 57–8
  spicy Egyptian bean (GF/DF) 65–6
  South Indian egg & coconut curry (GF)
  108–9
  South Indian mango curry (GF) 106–7
  South Indian tofu & mushroom curry (GF/
  DF) 110–11

soy sauce 35
Spanish stir-fry with cumin-yogurt sauce (GF) 72–3
spiced gazpacho with lemony egg (GF/DF) 57–8
spiced pickled onions (GF/DF) 192
spices 35
spicy Egyptian bean soup (GF/DF) 65–6
spicy Mexican bean flatbread 76
spicy palm heart & egg salad (GF/DF) 47–8
spinach, creamy spiked (GF) 136–7
stews
  green gumbo with Parmesan (DF) 94–5
  sweet & sour bean & beetroot (GF/DF) 92–3
stir-fry
  Spanish stir-fry with cumin-yogurt sauce (GF) 72–3
  with tofu (GF/DF) 71–2
strawberry vanilla porridge (DF) 163
sunflower seeds
  micro-broccoli salad with sweet seed clusters & egg (GF/DF) 54–5
swede
  Thai salad wraps with chargrilled tofu (GF/DF) 49–50
sweet & sour bean & beetroot stew (GF/DF) 92–3
sweet & sour tofu & pineapple (GF/DF) 97–8
sweet lentil cabbage wraps (GF/DF) 82–3
sweet potato & palm heart casserole (GF/DF) 104–5
sweetcorn, creamy chilli sweetcorn frittata (GF) 178–9
sweeteners 36

tabbouleh, raw cauliflower & feta (GF/DF) 44–5
tagine, vegetable & chickpea (GF/DF) 90–1
tea 198–9
  fridge 199
  iced almond tea cooler (GF/DF) 204
tempeh
  roasted tempeh with crisp capers (GF/DF) 144–5
teriyaki tofu & roasted broccoli (GF/DF) 99–100
Thai salad wraps with chargrilled tofu (GF/DF) 49–50
three-tomato & mozzarella flatbread 74–5
tofu 31–2
  hot and sour tofu bowl (GF/DF) 96–7
  meaty tofu mini-fillets (GF/DF) 139–40
  miso aubergine & tofu with red cabbage salad (GF/DF) 55–6
  miso noodle bowl (GF/DF) 69–70
  piquant marinade for (GF/DF) 140–1
  smoky BBQ marinade for (GF/DF) 142–3
  South Indian tofu & mushroom curry (GF/DF) 110–11
  stir-fry with (GF/DF) 71–2
  sweet & sour tofu & pineapple (GF/DF) 97–8
  teriyaki tofu & roasted broccoli (GF/DF) 99–100
  Thai salad wraps with chargrilled (GF/DF) 49–50
tomatoes 28
  almond & tomato sauce (GF/DF) 155–6
  dill & garlic tomatoes on cheese toast 170
  frozen Virgin Mary pops (GF/DF) 193
  Greek-style butterbeans with herbs & (GF/DF) 88–9

Mexican scramble (GF) 176
Napoli sauce (GF/DF) 151–2
pappa al pomodoro (DF) 68–9
three-tomato & mozzarella flatbread 74–5
tortilla, breakfast burrito 182–3
turnips
  Thai salad wraps with chargrilled tofu (GF/
    DF) 49–50

vanilla, strawberry vanilla porridge (DF) 163
vegetable stock 34
vegetable(s)
  & chickpea tagine (GF/DF) 90–1
  cooking 27
  marinated crudités (GF/DF) 187–8
  preparing 27
  selecting 26
  storing 27
vinegars 35

walnuts
  cold cucumber soup with (GF) 59–60
  Georgian-style beans in walnut &
    coriander sauce (GF/DF) 86–7
  green lightning salsa (GF/DF) 146–7
water, flavoured 199
water chestnuts, marinated water (GF/DF)
  189
wraps
  breakfast burrito 182–3
  spicy Mexican bean flatbread 76
  sweet lentil cabbage (GF/DF) 82–3
  Thai salad wraps with chargrilled tofu (GF/
    DF) 49–50
  three-tomato & mozzarella flatbread 74–5

xanthan gum 37, 164

yogurt
  cold cucumber soup with walnuts (GF)
    59–60
  creamy paprika mushrooms (GF) 80–1
  creamy sesame sauce (GF) 156–7
  creamy spiked spinach (GF) 136–7
  cumin-yogurt dressing 51–2
  light ranch dip (GF) 191
  Spanish stir-fry with cumin-yogurt sauce
    (GF) 72–3

FOR JUSTIN

ACKNOWLEDGEMENTS

Heart-felt thanks to the amazing Emily Preece-Morrison for running with this idea and for your continuing support, enthusiasm and meticulous execution.

Thank you Maggie Ramsay – your editorial talents are off the charts and it was a blessing to have your dedication and reassurance.

Anita Bean, thanks so much for your thorough analysis and invaluable advice over the course of this project.

Georgina Hewitt, thanks for applying your awesome design skills and bringing beauty to this little volume. Thanks also to Welmoet Wartena and Laura Brodie for your great work, and to Claire Winfield for the striking cover photo.

Thanks to my dear friend Ben Gill – you planted the seed that made me curious about fasting, which led me ultimately to a positive life change, and now this book.

Massive gratitude to Dr Michael Mosley, for creating the documentary which convinced me to commit to 5:2, and for instigating a diet revolution that is improving countless lives across the globe.

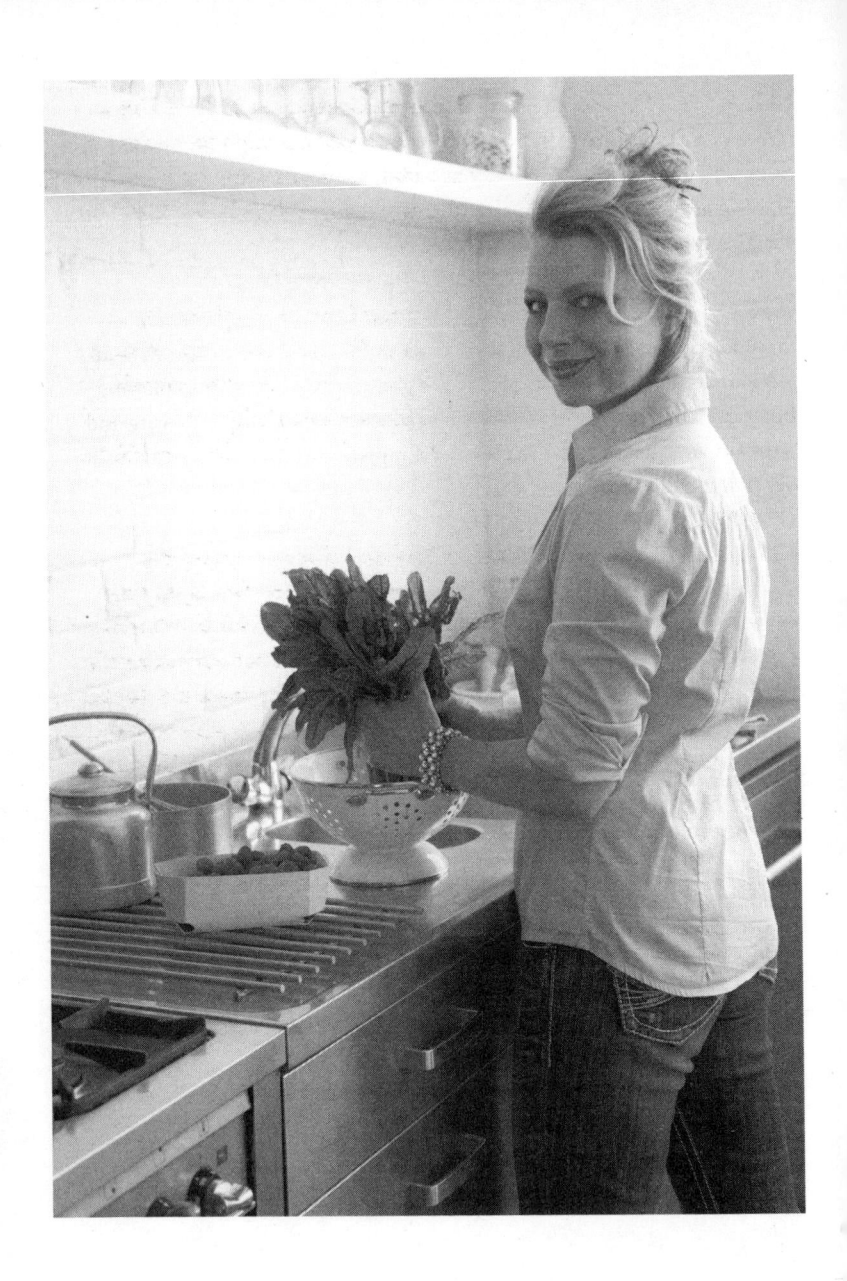

CELIA BROOKS moved to London from Colorado in 1989 seeking a career as a theatre director, but swiftly developed a passion for cooking and changed tack. She forged a career as a chef, food writer and businesswoman. Starting as a private chef for film director Stanley Kubrick and family, she went on to author several cookbooks.

Celia created her highly successful food tour business, Gastrotours, in 2002, as a platform to share her passion. She connects people with an array of artisan foods around London's gastronomic hotspots, including Borough Market and Portobello. Her extensive knowledge, curiosity and constant engagement with markets and ingredients have firmly established her as a top food expert.

Celia has had eight cookbooks published worldwide, including the recently updated and re-released *Low-Carb and Gluten-Free Vegetarian*, and numerous journalistic accomplishments, with columns for *The Times*, *BBC Good Food Magazine* and *The Evening Standard*. She currently writes for the Borough Market blog and the market's resident magazine, *Market Life*. She has also made multiple TV appearances. Her cooking style is fundamentally vegetarian, and she is also known as "The New Urban Farmer", writing about growing to eat, based on her experience tending her London allotment.

Find out more at *www.celiabrooksbrown.com* and *5-2veg.tumblr.com* or follow Celia on Twitter *@celiabb*